D0428235

Anxiety-Free Kids

Anxiety- Free Kids

Second Edition

An Interactive Guide for Parents and Children

Bonnie Zucker, Psy.D.

Illustrated by David Parker

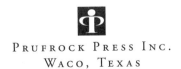

PRUFROCK PRESS INC.
WACO, TEXAS

Library of Congress catalog information
currently on file with the publisher.

Edited by Lacy Compton

Cover design by Raquel Trevino and layout design by Allegra Denbo

ISBN-13: 978-1-61821-561-1

Prufrock Press Inc.
P.O. Box 8813
Waco, TX 76714-8813
Phone: (800) 998-2208
Fax: (800) 240-0333
http://www.prufrock.com

I dedicate this to my husband, Brian, and our two radiant sons, Isaac and Todd. You three are my everything, and you bring me unimaginable joy. Your love is the greatest of all gifts.

And to my Mother, who taught me my two greatest lessons: how to love and how to be compassionate.

Table of Contents

Acknowledgements ix

Preface to the Second Edition xiii

Welcome to *Anxiety-Free Kids* xv

Introduction: *How to Use This Book* 1

A Note for Your Child's Therapist 3

CHAPTER 1
Anxiety: *What It Is and What to Do About It* 5

CHAPTER 2
Making Your Team and Team Goals 31

CHAPTER 3
Relaxing the Body 47

CHAPTER 4
Conquer Your Worries 71

CHAPTER 5
Changing Your Thoughts 89

CHAPTER 6
Changing Your Behaviors: *Facing Your Fears* 107

CHAPTER 7
Keep Facing Your Fears and Build Confidence 117

CHAPTER 8
Lessons Learned: *Celebrate Yourself* 129

CHAPTER 9
Motivating Your Child 135

CHAPTER 10
Special Sections 145

CHAPTER 11
Anxiety at Bedtime: *Improving Sleep Behavior* 181

CHAPTER 12
Parenting Your Anxious Child: *Adopting a Resilience Mindset* . . . 189

References 197

Resources for Parents 201

Appendix A: *Overview of the Program* 209

Appendix B: *Thinking Errors Quick Reference Page* 211

About the Author 213

ANXIETY-FREE KIDS:
"For Kids Only" Companion Guide 217

Acknowledgements

WRITING this book, and its revision, has been an incredibly rewarding experience. In 1998, I discovered my love for treating anxiety disorders. Since that time, I have had the privilege of helping many children and adults who entrusted me with their well-being. They have taught me so much about life from their ability to grow and achieve psychological freedom. Their resilience and strength are extraordinarily impressive. Their progress is at the root of my motivation to write this book. It is my hope that it inspires the same growth in others.

The mentors and colleagues who have shown unending confidence in me have allowed me to become a stronger clinician. Dr. Bernard Vittone and Dr. Mary Alvord are chief among them. A special thank you to Dr. Vittone for sharing his expertise in the medication portion of the parent book. Drs. Rudy Bauer, Bill Lee, and Bill Stixrud have contributed to my growth, both personally and professionally. A special thank you to Dr. John McPherrin, who taught me how to be authentic and real with clients. I cannot thank Rich Weinfeld enough for connecting me with Prufrock, and for his continued enthusiasm. Finally, I want to thank Dr. Harvey Parker, who is the reason why I became a psychologist. His warmth, compassionate nature, and mastery of cognitive behavioral therapy make him an extraordinary psychologist and a phenomenal person.

Thank you to Dr. Judith Rapoport and Dr. Golda Ginsburg for their willingness to review and support this book. Their dedication to childhood anxiety disorders and expertise in the field is exceptional. I am honored by their endorsement of this book.

Lacy Compton, my editor at Prufrock, has been a pleasure to work with from the beginning. Her enthusiasm for this project and her superb skill as an editor shaped this book (and its previous version) in wonderful ways. I am extremely grateful for her contributions and guidance.

My husband, Brian, has shared my passion for this project and has supported me at every level. He has demonstrated unconditional belief in me and my work as a psychologist, and has been patient and understanding during the many times I have needed to "go and write." Brian, and our little loves, Isaac and Todd, fill my life with love and warmth, and this makes me a better person in every way, including in my role as a clinician.

My mother was a constant source of love and encouragement throughout my life. The direction she provided, the confidence and security she gave, and the model of strength and goodness she demonstrated were instrumental in helping me to carve my own path in life and to become the person I am today. She always cheered me on and taught me how to be resilient; although she is no longer here to see the second edition of this book, she loved the first edition and it was a great source of pride for her.

I will forever be grateful for the sisterhood and best friendship that I have shared with Emily Celler. Her love and unfailing support mean more to me than she could ever fully realize. A special thank you to Ilene, Norm, Lisa, Scott, and Shawn, who have always celebrated my achievements with enthusiasm and pride.

Finally, I am influenced every day by the light and warmth of several individuals whose love constantly surrounds me though they are no longer here. My father's memory brings me strength.

The way he lived his life motivates me to succeed and work hard, and to be unwaveringly ethical. My stepfather, Irv, taught me how to live in awareness. His capacity for equality consciousness has influenced me in immeasurable ways. Most of all, his generosity of spirit and unconditional love have impacted me greatly. My grandparents, Ruth and Ben, nurtured me and nourished me with love and sweetness and modeled how to live a good and honorable life. These influences shine brightly in my life.

Preface to the Second Edition

IN the 9 years that have passed since writing this book, I have had the privilege of treating hundreds more children with anxiety. I get to go to "work" every day and witness the growth and transformation of so many children and teens as they look deeply within themselves and find the courage and strength to face their fears, negotiate a new relationship with their thoughts, and create a new life of liberation and freedom. In doing so, I have learned so much more about anxiety and how it is overcome. I have become a better clinician, more knowledgeable, and even more confident in the power of cognitive-behavioral therapy. These insights and knowledge are reflected in this second edition.

In addition to a revised first edition, I have added two additional chapters: one on sleep and one on how to best parent a child with anxiety. Given how many kids have trouble falling asleep on their own in their own beds, or falling asleep in general, and how many parents struggle to help their children with this issue, a chapter on the subject seemed necessary. My work with anxious children always involves working with their parent(s). Being an effective parent to a child with anxiety not only supports the child in overcoming it, but facilitates more growth in the parents; by becoming successful in their parenting role around the anxiety, they develop more confidence and competence as parents in general.

Welcome to
Anxiety-Free Kids

WELCOME to *Anxiety-Free Kids: An Interactive Guide for Parents and Children* (2nd ed.). This book features a unique companion-book approach, offering both an information book for parents and a tear-out workbook for kids. Congratulations on the selection of this book's program to help your child overcome his or her anxieties, fears, and worrying behavior. It is a sign of resourcefulness and good parenting to take this step to assist your child in improving his or her experience in life, including his or her self-confidence and overall feeling of safety. This program is based on the cognitive-behavioral therapy (CBT) approach to treating anxiety disorders and it involves teaching strategies and techniques to overcome anxiety. CBT is problem-focused and solution-oriented and considers anxiety to have three components: physiological reactions, faulty and irrational thoughts, and avoidance or other nervous behaviors. It goes beyond figuring out the *causes* of the anxiety and primarily focuses on how to treat it. CBT is proactive and includes developing a detailed plan for overcoming the three parts of anxiety.

The need for a companion-book approach, including a book for the child and a parallel book for his or her parent(s), is based on the belief that the most comprehensive approach to treating a child's problem involves integrating the system in which the child lives. The field of psychology calls this a *family systems approach*, and research shows that it is a very effective way of treating the child's problem. By this, I mean that your child can use your help, but your child will do the bulk of the work while you will offer guidance, direction, encouragement, and most importantly, continuous support and praise. In addition, your insights into your child's thoughts and behaviors will be invaluable in helping him or her complete the necessary steps to overcoming anxiety and feeling better. Although other books may have a "companion" book for the child, no other series to date is designed to be read simultaneously by parent and child. The chapters in each book are paired together and address the same topic; thus, they parallel each other and are to be read separately, but together. The tear-out companion guide for kids begins immediately after your parent book begins. Simply remove the perforated pages from this book and staple each chapter together for your child. It is recommended that you and your child read and discuss one chapter at a time, and that each chapter is fully understood by your child before moving on to the next one. Also, the chapters should be read in order, without skipping any chapters.

Some children also have therapists (psychologists, psychiatrists, social workers, or professional counselors) or may begin seeing one at some point. This program is intended to be all you need to help your child overcome anxiety; however, some parents will find that their child requires more than this program. If professional help is sought, this program will be an excellent supplement to your child's work with a therapist, and will guide the therapist on how to treat the anxiety from a CBT perspective. For this reason I have included the section after the Introduction entitled "A Note for Your Therapist."

All of the chapters include exercises at the end for you and your child to complete together. Some of these exercises include discussion topics and questions, while others include projects or activities. These exercises are essential in order to get the most out of the program. Generally, it is recommended that you and your child schedule time together once a week to discuss what you have read and to work on the activities. I encourage you to make these meetings as enjoyable as possible for your child (e.g., they can be outdoors in a park, at a favorite restaurant, or followed by a movie). Many children find such one-on-one time with parents quite valuable. If your child sees a therapist, your child should do the exercises with the therapist; you should receive feedback from the therapist about the exercises at each therapy session and review the exercises with your child after the session.

Although the word *parent* is used throughout each book, two parents or caregivers can read the chapters and the child can work with as many adults as desired on the activities/discussion exercises. This book is designed to be read by caretakers—and this includes stepparents, grandparents, foster parents, aunts, uncles, and so forth—however, for simplicity, I will refer to the reader as "parent," because this represents the most common situation. Finally, I will switch between male and female pronouns for the purpose of easy reading.

Best of luck,
Dr. Bonnie Zucker

Introduction

How to Use This Book

BEFORE we get started, let me tell you a little about how this program works. You and your child will read your respective books at the same time. The pages of the "For Kids Only Companion Guide" are perforated and easy to tear out. It is best to pull out and staple or clip together each chapter individually, and then present the chapters to your child one at a time to help him or her manage the task of reading the book. The chapters are matched up with one another and the content generally is the same, covering the same topics and issues. For example, Chapter 1 in both books is an introduction to anxiety. Your chapters typically will be longer and include additional information on how you can best assist your child through this program.

At the end of each chapter, there is an exercise designed to be completed together by you and your child. The exercises are explained in both books, but your book also contains recommendations on how to complete the exercises and get the most out of them, including how to make it a fun experience for you and your child. The exercises are an integral part of the program and are essential to its success. Appendix A provides an overview of the program in table form and this allows you and your child to check off when each chapter and exercise has been completed.

Your child's book explains that words like *parents, mom,* and *dad* are used interchangeably to describe who is completing this program with him or her, yet clarifies that other caring adults can use it too.

Finally, although I would like to think that children will be excited to read this book and be motivated solely by the prospect of feeling better, sometimes a little prompting is necessary. This may involve rewarding your child for each chapter he or she reads or for each exercise the two of you complete. I do not encourage paying your child for reading this book. However, I see nothing wrong with rewarding him or her with a privilege, such as computer time or play time or allowing him or her to choose a small prize from a "reward treasure chest" (get a box, make a personalized label for it, such as "Brian's Box of Bonuses," and fill it with small toys from the dollar store, bubble gum, homemade coupons for renting a movie of his or her choice, and so forth). In the end, the most important thing is that the child reads the chapters and completes the exercises. As always, verbal praise is of utmost importance, and once we get to the exposure phase, your child is going to need a great deal of it.

OK, let's get started!

DON'T FORGET!

1. Tear out the "For Kids Only Companion Guide" and staple or clip each chapter together.
2. Give your child one chapter at a time. Read your respective chapters at the same time.
3. Complete the exercise at the end of each chapter together.
4. Use rewards if necessary.

A Note for Your Child's Therapist

WELCOME to *Anxiety-Free Kids*! This two-book companion approach offers an excellent guide for you, your child client, and the child's family. I designed this book to be used either as a self-help book or as a supplement to the child's therapy. Using a cognitive-behavioral therapy (CBT) framework, the child and his parent are directed through the various steps to overcoming the child's anxiety. Six anxiety disorders are addressed: generalized anxiety disorder, separation anxiety disorder, social anxiety disorder, specific phobia, obsessive-compulsive disorder, and panic disorder. The CBT can be integrated into whatever other work you are doing, or orientation you are taking, with the child.

The child and parent read eight chapters together and then the parent's section includes four additional chapters. Each chapter includes an exercise at the end. It is my recommendation that you complete the exercises with the child during your session time (e.g., make self-talk note cards with him or her in the session). You may or may not choose to include parents in the process of completing the exercises; at minimum, parents should be asked to contribute examples of the child's anxious and avoidance behaviors and should receive feedback on the exercises and what was accomplished in the session. I also highly recommend that you help the child learn the thinking errors and identify which ones she uses most often when she is anxious. Finally, should you feel the child would benefit from Attention Training Technique (described in Chapter 10 under OCD), the script for this is available in Adrian Wells's 2011 book (see reference section).

Best of luck,
Dr. Bonnie Zucker

CHAPTER

1

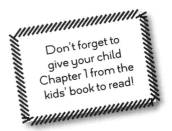

Don't forget to give your child Chapter 1 from the kids' book to read!

Anxiety

What It Is and What to Do About It

Ten-year-old Kimberly worries a lot. She worries about her homework, her dog, her house, and what other kids think about her. Kimberly has a hard time adjusting to unexpected changes. Last week when her mom picked her up from school and told her about her dentist appointment, Kimberly had a meltdown and became very upset because Mom didn't tell her about it the day before. The appointment had to be rescheduled. When doing homework, Kimberly often gets very nervous about not having enough time to finish it, even though it usually takes about an hour, and sometimes becomes so stressed that she cannot concentrate or organize her thoughts. She worries that someone will break into her house and possibly kidnap her, and each time she approaches her house, her heart starts to beat fast. For this reason, Kimberly refuses to be the first person to walk into the house and has her mom or dad go in first and check that no one has broken in. Kimberly also checks on her dog many times each day to make sure he is OK and didn't run out of the house. Kimberly gets a lot of stomachaches and headaches from all of her worrying.

KIMBERLY, and many children like her, suffers from an anxiety disorder. Her childhood is filled with worries and feelings of uneasiness. Kimberly's parents struggle to make her feel calm and comfortable and feel at a loss of what to do to help her. If your child has anxiety like Kimberly, or has a different type of anxiety, then this book is for you. You and your child will receive guidance on how to become aware of what his anxiety symptoms are and how they can be addressed and overcome in a step-by-step fashion. You will soon discover that you and your child don't need to be organized and controlled by anxiety. You and your child will overcome this and will be liberated.

In this chapter, your child will learn the following:

1. common symptoms of anxiety,
2. how to differentiate normal versus problematic anxiety,
3. the three parts of anxiety, and
4. how to address each of the three parts of anxiety.

These topics will be addressed in this chapter, and the exercise that you will complete with your child after you each read Chapter 1 of your respective books will be reviewed. This chapter also will include descriptions of the different anxiety disorders, an explanation of the cognitive-behavioral therapy (CBT) approach to treating anxiety disorders, how best to use this program with your child and what to say to him or her when implementing it, and advice on determining if your child requires professional help and/or medication.

Anxiety: Its Symptoms and Disorders

Anxiety is the experience of feeling nervous, worried, scared, or afraid, and is the opposite of feeling relaxed. All children and adults feel anxious at times. Sometimes anxiety arises as a result of an event, such as when you are driving and almost hit the car in front of you. Sometimes it appears out of the blue. Our capacity for anxiety is a survival mechanism that allows us to react quickly in a threatening situation by providing a physical reaction known as the "flight or fight" response. In addition, anxiety can be a motivator and can help us get things done in a timely manner. For example, the anxiety associated with having to pass a test serves as a motivator for studying for it.

Anxiety involves three parts: physiological feelings (body), thoughts, and behavior. Typically, the behavior associated with anxiety is avoidance. When children and adults avoid anxiety-provoking situations, such avoidance breeds self-doubt. Over time, the repetitive practice of self-doubting impacts and even damages one's self-esteem.

The diagram in Figure 1 is included in your child's chapter to help him or her conceptualize the three parts of anxiety.

In order to understand and treat anxiety, we need to understand and address the three parts. Each part will be discussed in greater detail in later chapters. Common physical (*body*) symptoms of anxiety are:

- ▶ rapid heart rate,
- ▶ shallow breathing,
- ▶ muscle tension,
- ▶ sweating,
- ▶ restlessness,
- ▶ difficulty swallowing,
- ▶ choking sensations,
- ▶ dizziness,
- ▶ stomachaches,
- ▶ shaking, and
- ▶ feeling detached from one's body or from reality.

Somatic complaints are physical symptoms that are psychological in nature (have no organic or medical cause) and include stomachaches, headaches, and general aches and pains. If your child displays what appear to be somatic complaints, I recommend that he or she receive a comprehensive physical exam to rule out any underlying physical problem even though you may feel the cause is psychological.

The cognitive (or *thoughts*) part of anxiety includes the following: worries, thinking errors, negative self-talk, and a perceived irrational threat. Anxious children often will use "what if's" when

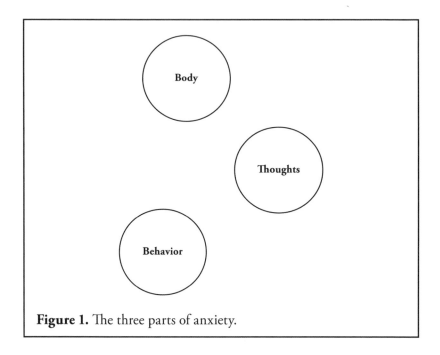

Figure 1. The three parts of anxiety.

they worry about bad things happening to them or to their parents or loved ones. Worries also may center on performance in social situations, such as test anxiety and social anxiety. Examples of thinking errors, also known as cognitive distortions, include:

- "Other kids will laugh at me if I raise my hand and give the wrong answer,"
- "I should get all A's in school. Getting a B means that I am a failure,"
- "It happened to her so it will happen to me," and
- "What if someone breaks in and hurts us?"

As mentioned above, the *behavior* part of anxiety typically includes avoidance behavior. However, if the child does not avoid the anxiety-provoking situation, he or she will endure it with extreme distress. Examples of avoidance include:

- not going near the feared object (dogs, injections);

▶ refusing to separate from Mom or Dad;

▶ not sleeping alone;

▶ refusing to go over to a friend's house for a sleepover; and

▶ refusing to go to school.

Children with anxiety often display nervous behaviors, such as seeking reassurance (asking a parent or caregiver to tell them that they will be OK), checking behaviors (e.g., checking that doors are locked, checking that parents are OK), picking/pulling behaviors, crying, freezing up, and having a meltdown or tantrum.

Now let's look at the three parts again, taking into account what each entails. (See Figure 2.)

Anxiety goes from being "normal" to being a problem or disorder in need of treatment when it causes a significant interference in the child's life. This is the key factor in determining if your child needs help in dealing with her anxiety. If the anxiety interferes with your child's academic or social performance (e.g., it prevents your child from going to school, birthday parties, or sleepovers, or from sleeping alone at night, or if it renders her unable to concentrate at school due to focusing on worries), or interferes with your child's ability to enjoy life or feel good about herself (e.g., daily stomachaches or headaches, persistent worry, negative self-image), this is a good indication that her anxiety has become a disorder. A fear of something becomes a phobia when it involves avoidance of the feared object or situation *or* if exposure to the feared object or situation is endured with extreme distress and causes a significant impairment in her life.

Anxiety Disorders

Anxiety disorders are the most common form of psychological disorders in children and adults. Anxiety disorders occur in one in eight children (Anxiety Disorder Association of America, n.d.) and the lifetime prevalence of anxiety disorders in children

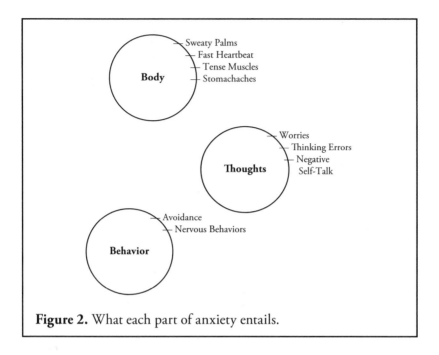

Figure 2. What each part of anxiety entails.

aged 13–18 is 25% (Merikangas et al., n.d.). Research has demonstrated that an untreated anxiety disorder in childhood often persists into adulthood. Anxiety is considered to be an internalizing disorder, meaning that its symptoms are not always evident from the perspective of an outsider. This is in contrast with externalizing disorders, such as disruptive or aggressive behaviors, which are hard to miss. It also is important to note that anxiety disorders (specifically generalized anxiety disorder) and Attention Deficit/Hyperactivity Disorder (ADHD) have symptoms that overlap. For example, restlessness, difficulty concentrating, difficulty sustaining focus, and one's mind going blank are all symptoms of both disorders. Consider the difficulty associated with trying to balance your checkbook while fearing that at any moment, someone will break into your house and harm you. Thus, making a differential diagnosis is very important, as the treatments are different. In particular, the medication treatment typically used for ADHD (stimulant medication such as Ritalin and Adderall) may impair the treatment of anxiety disorders, as these medications can result in an increase in anxiety symptoms.

Several different anxiety disorders are listed in the American Psychological Association's (2013) *Diagnostic and Statistical Manual of Mental Disorders*, fifth edition (DSM-5; the Bible of psychiatric disorders). When an individual meets the criteria for one disorder and for another disorder, this is called *comorbidity*. The most common comorbid disorder for an anxiety disorder is another anxiety disorder, but many children also experience depression. In addition, children with other diagnoses can have a comorbid anxiety disorder; for example, a National Institute of Mental Health (NIMH; Jensen et al., 2001) study found that about 30%–35% of children with ADHD have an existing anxiety disorder (CHADD, n.d.).

The six disorders that I most often see in children include:

▸ generalized anxiety disorder (GAD),
▸ separation anxiety disorder (SAD),
▸ social anxiety disorder (SoP),
▸ specific phobia (SP),
▸ obsessive-compulsive disorder (OCD), and
▸ panic disorder (PD).

In the DSM-V, OCD, which was previously classified as an anxiety disorder, became its own category, along with other disorders including hoarding disorder and trichotillomania (hair pulling), now called Obsessive-Compulsive and Related Disorders. Unlike previous versions of the DSM, the DSM-V places categories of related conditions sequentially, so the Obsessive-Compulsive category naturally follows the Anxiety Disorders category, illustrating that OCD is related to Anxiety Disorders. Given that children with OCD often experience and present with anxiety, I have continued to include OCD in this book's second edition.

Each disorder is discussed in greater detail in Chapter 10, but a brief overview of the disorders below should help you as you work with your child. Remember that it also may be beneficial to read more about the disorder you suspect your child may have by turning to Chapter 10 before beginning the program. I provide guidance specific to the particular anxiety or issue your child is experiencing; reading Chapter 10 should be considered just as pertinent as Chapters 1–8 in helping your child through this program.

Generalized anxiety disorder (GAD) is characterized by excessive worry that occurs more days than not for at least 6 months and is difficult to contain. The symptoms include restlessness, being easily fatigued, difficulty concentrating, irritability, muscle tension, sleep disturbance, and physical complaints.

Separation anxiety disorder (SAD) involves excessive distress when the child is separated from home or from attachment figures or when separation is anticipated. The child often worries about harm befalling major attachment figures, like parents, and may refuse to go to school or elsewhere in efforts to avoid separation. Children with SAD often refuse to sleep in their own beds or without their parent(s) present and may exhibit physical symptoms or complaints when separation occurs or is anticipated.

Social anxiety disorder (SoP) is the fear of social or performance situations in which the child will be exposed to unfamiliar people or possible scrutiny by others. A child with social anxiety fears that he or she will act in a way that will be embarrassing or humiliating and tends to believe that there is a great likelihood that a negative event or outcome will occur in social or performance situations.

Specific phobias (SP) are pretty easy to identify. This is what people generally think of when they say someone has a phobia. Specific phobias involve marked and persistent fear that is excessive or unreasonable and occurs in the presence of, anticipation of, or exposure to a specific object or situation. Exposure to the phobic situation is either avoided or endured with extreme distress. The DSM-5 lists five subtypes of specific phobias: animal, natural environment (storms, heights, water), blood-injection-injury type, situational (flying, elevators, enclosed places), and other.

Obsessive-compulsive disorder (OCD) is characterized by the presence of obsessions or compulsions, but usually both occur. Obsessions are intrusive thoughts, images, or impulses. For example, contamination fears, harm to others, and symmetry urges (everything needs to be perfectly ordered and aligned) are all obsessions. Compulsions or rituals are repetitive intentional behaviors or mental acts performed in response to an obsession. For example, washing, checking, touching in a certain way, counting, and ordering all are compulsions or rituals. The compulsions are performed in order to reduce the anxiety caused by obsessions. To meet the criteria for OCD, the symptoms must cause distress and must either be time-consuming (taking at least one hour a day) or cause a significant interference with the child's normal routine, academic functioning, or social interaction.

Finally, *panic disorder* (PD) includes the presence of panic attacks and a fear of having additional panic attacks. Situations in which the child is afraid of having an attack often are avoided. A panic attack is a terrifying experience in which the individual is consumed with at least four of the following symptoms (listed in the DSM-5), most of which are experienced as physical in nature:

1. palpitations, pounding heart, or accelerated heart rate;
2. sweating;
3. trembling or shaking;
4. sensations of shortness of breath or smothering;
5. feeling of choking;
6. chest pain or discomfort;
7. nausea or abdominal distress;
8. feeling dizzy, unsteady, lightheaded, or faint;
9. de-realization (feelings of unreality) or depersonalization (being detached from oneself);
10. fear of losing control or going crazy;
11. fear of dying;
12. paresthesias (numbness or tingling sensations); or
13. chills or hot flushes.

In order to become familiar with the different anxiety disorders, try to identify which anxiety disorder is described in the six examples listed below.

▶ At the age of 6, James was in his backyard helping his father pull weeds from the garden. As he pulled out one large weed, a garden snake jumped out at him and landed on his stomach before falling to the ground. After this experience, James became afraid of snakes. He began to worry about encountering a snake. Whenever he was outdoors, he would be on guard looking for snakes. If he heard an animal moving in the bushes, he would run away, fearing that it was a snake. As years passed, James's fear grew and grew. When he watched a scene from one of the *Harry Potter* movies that had a snake in it, he became terrified. He refused to go to his friend's house because the friend kept a snake as a pet. James even avoided eating cucumbers as they reminded him of snakes! Sometimes James would even feel sick to his stomach just thinking of snakes, and wouldn't eat spaghetti or other foods that were "snake-like." He came in for therapy at the age of 12 as his symptoms were continuing to get worse.

▶ One night before bed, Emily was in her room when she suddenly felt like she was choking, and couldn't breathe. It seemed to come out of nowhere. She immediately ran to get her mother and told her mother what was happening, and that she thought she could be dying. Her heart was pounding, she felt dizzy, and began to feel a flush of hot and then cold running through her body. As this was happening, she worried about what was happening to her, and felt like it wasn't real. This feeling made her even more afraid and she began sobbing as her mother held her and rubbed her back. Eventually, Emily was able to catch her breath and calm down, though she still felt shaky for a few more hours. The next night as she was getting ready for bed, Emily told her mother that she worried it would happen again. She decided not to go to a sleepover party the next weekend because she did not want to go through this again when she was not in the comfort of her own home and with her family.

▶ Billy was a very bright 9-year-old with a phenomenal imagination. He spent his time designing very sophisticated and creative games and was always happy when he worked on his games. Despite being so bright, Billy had a learning disability and took a very long time to do writing assignments at school. Some of his teachers did not understand that he had a learning disability and would punish him for not having all his work done. At times, he even had to stay in from recess to finish his work. This made Billy feel very uncomfortable and embarrassed. He began to worry about getting in trouble and having to stay back. As a result, Billy would daydream and had trouble focusing on his work. He had very tense muscles, found it difficult to go to sleep, and often would stay up most of the night worrying. Billy complained to his mother and father about headaches and feeling tired. His worry interfered with his ability to concentrate and focus on his schoolwork. Sometimes he would be so worried that he would not want to go to school.

▶ Carlos was a responsible, bright, and athletic 12-year-old with lots of friends. His parents described him as shy and quiet, but well-liked by others. Carlos reported that he felt very uncomfortable at school, especially during class and basketball games. In particular, he worried that he would speak in class and say something "stupid," and that others would laugh at him. He worried so much that he never raised his hand and dreaded the times that a teacher called on him. Carlos also worried that he would forget about a test or quiz and that he would fail and the teacher would get mad at him. When playing basketball, he was terrified that he would make a mistake and embarrass himself. As a result, he often missed basketball games.

▶ Ten-year-old Ruth spent a lot of time worrying that she would get sick. Specifically, she thought that she would get sick by getting germs from others. When at a sleepover, Ruth refused to eat chips out of a bowl that others had touched. She never ate anything homemade, especially baked goods, or anything from the school cafeteria. Using public bathrooms was so uncomfortable for her that she often "held it" until she got home. When she did use public bathrooms, she did her best not to touch anything there—she used her foot to flush the toilet and used paper towels or her sleeve to touch the faucet and door handles. If Ruth accidentally touched anything in the bathroom, even the walls of the stall, she would insist that her mother wash her clothes immediately once they got home. She wanted her mom to wash everything twice, to make sure the germs were gone. Even though she didn't really know why she was so afraid of germs, sometimes she would become so distressed about getting germs on her that she would stay at home in her room all day.

▶ Thelma became very anxious when she would separate from her mother. It even bothered her if her mother went out to the front of the house to take out the trash. In public places, Thelma refused to go to the bathroom alone and insisted that someone went with her. At home, she always left the bathroom door wide open. She worried that something bad would happen to her or to her mother. When her mother left the room, she would sing to Thelma so Thelma would know which room her mother was in at all times. If her mother would go out to art class, Thelma would get very sick and many times, she would vomit. Her mother felt so bad about this that she decided to bring Thelma with her to art class.

Answers: James meets the criteria for a specific phobia; Emily has panic disorder; Billy has generalized anxiety disorder; Carlos has social anxiety disorder; Ruth has obsessive-compulsive disorder; and Thelma has separation anxiety disorder.

What to Do About It: Cognitive-Behavioral Therapy

Cognitive-behavioral therapy (CBT) is the most empirically supported approach in the treatment of anxiety disorders in children and adults. This means that the research on the different types of therapies used to treat anxiety disorders has shown that the cognitive-behavioral approach is the most effective. In all honesty, I love it. We all have our passions, and you may think it is a little odd that mine is CBT, but it really is *that* good! It is problem-focused and solution-oriented, practical, short-term (e.g., an average of 12–16 sessions), provides the client with useful coping strategies and techniques, and it helps children change their thinking patterns that not only help them with their anxiety now, but theoretically can serve to prevent problems from developing in the future (many anxieties develop out of and worsen from thinking errors/ irrational thinking, and the resulting impact on behavior, which is avoidance). In addition, by challenging one's thinking patterns, CBT can result in a significant improvement in one's self-esteem and self-confidence (e.g., by challenging the distorted thinking and guiding the child in facing his fears).

Although other therapies can be helpful, research consistently finds that CBT is the best approach to effectively treating anxiety in children and adults (Christophersen & Mortweet, 2001; Hollon, Stewart, & Strunk, 2006; Otte, 2011; Sburlati, Lyneham, Schniering, & Rapee, 2014). I believe this is largely due to CBT's focus on facing fears and providing strategies and techniques for doing so. Other approaches, such as classic psychoanalytic therapy, are less structured, less directive, and often do not involve the teaching of strategies or techniques. Rather, the psychoanalytic approach is aimed at understanding the causes of the anxiety disorder, including the unconscious experience of the child. In my view, this is unhelpful for a child with anxiety who needs direction and techniques to cope with his symptoms and to challenge avoidance behavior.

So, what is CBT anyway? Well, you already have been introduced to the cognitive-behavioral understanding that anxiety involves three parts: physiological (body symptoms), cognition (thoughts), and behavior. CBT considers the connection between thoughts and feelings, and the philosophy is, you can change the way you feel by changing the way you think. This point is very important to remember when helping your child with his or her anxiety: If we can change the way we *think*, we can change the way we *feel*. So, if we think differently, we can reduce our feelings of anxiety. In terms of thinking patterns, CBT explains that individuals with anxiety make thinking errors (I refer to them as *thinking mistakes* in your child's book) and that these errors cause, maintain, and strengthen the anxiety. CBT teaches the child to replace these thinking errors with rational responses (reality-based, logical thoughts), a practice particularly helpful in addressing worries and phobias. Changing the way you think also involves altering one's inner dialogue or *self-talk*: changing negative thoughts to coping thoughts. It is also a goal for your child to change his relationship with his thoughts: to see the thoughts as just anxious thoughts that are better explained as being a symptom of anxiety rather than a thought deserving real consideration. In this edition, I have included guidance on how to practice detached mindfulness, a strategy from metacognitive therapy that has the goal of changing one's relationship to his or her thoughts (this is explained in detail in Chapter 5). CBT also helps decrease anxiety through practicing relaxation and calm breathing. Equally, if not more, important is working on the behaviors associated with anxiety, namely avoidance. The behavioral part of CBT explains that one's anxiety is maintained and strengthened by avoidance behaviors. To treat this, the child needs to be *systematically desensitized* (or gradually exposed) to the anxiety-provoking situations, starting with the ones that elicit the least anxiety and gradually moving up toward the ones that seem most frightening. This is consistent with the "face your fears" mentality. When the child is exposed to the anxiety-provoking situation, he or she will experience anxiety. However, if the child stays in the situation, the anxiety will begin to decrease. This process is called *habituation*. For example, if a child with a dog phobia spends one hour a day with different dogs, this child will get used to being with dogs and no longer will feel anxious around them. Then the child will begin to relax when he or she is around dogs, pairing together dogs and a relaxed feeling. In fact, it is the behavior change (facing your fears) that actually leads to overcoming the anxiety disorder. I love the saying: *Courage comes after slaying the dragon!* Your child will discover so much about his potential from facing his fears.

When treating anxiety, behavior change happens first and cognitive change (thought change) happens second. For example, with a dog phobia, the child will be near a dog and pet a dog before the worries (thoughts) about what the dog may do (e.g., bite) go away. With repeated behavior change, the thoughts eventually go away. The brain literally starts to experience the previously feared situation as neutral and unalarming.

Sounds pretty good, right? Well, the best part is that the program in this book is based on cognitive-behavioral theory and therapy. The techniques your child will learn to use to cope with anxiety and the exercises you will complete together all are rooted in CBT.

In order to effectively treat anxiety, all three parts must be addressed. Prior to considering each part, we need to talk about the importance of externalizing the anxiety. As discussed earlier, anxiety is an internalizing disorder, and children feel like the anxiety is a part of them. The goal is for this to shift so the child can view anxiety as something separate from him or her. One way to do this is to encourage your child to identify his or her worries and nervous feelings as anxiety. For instance, when you hear your child expressing separation worries, say to him: "That's the anxiety talking. When you feel worried about something bad happening to Mommy, it's the anxiety talking to you." In Chapter 4, you and your child will work together to make a list called, "When My Anxiety Talks, It Says . . ." The more you emphasize this, the easier it will be for your child to identify the symptoms of anxiety and to work toward overcoming them. Your child will learn that it's her against the anxiety or fear, and that each time she listens to the fear and avoids a situation, the fear wins and becomes stronger. One key component is helping your child understand that to beat the anxiety and win, he or she will need to learn that anxiety itself is not that scary. Although anxiety is uncomfortable, it is not dangerous. This logic is important to grasp and seems a bit counterintuitive. Because anxiety is unpleasant, we try to avoid it; however, in avoiding it, we become more anxious. You and your child will come to see that, in breaking the anxiety cycle, he will have to be able to tolerate some anxious experiences (e.g., when facing his fears). By tolerating, or "staying with" the anxiety, your child learns that the unpleasant sensations are manageable and the anxiety lessens as a result. Helping your child to understand the symptoms of his anxiety disorder and the principle of learning not to fear the anxiety will lay the foundation for facing his fears.

We will go through the three parts of anxiety (body, thoughts, and behavior) in order, starting with the body. You and your child will learn deep breathing, progressive muscle relaxation (PMR), guided imagery relaxation, mindfulness meditation, and yoga. For the thoughts component, your child will learn positive self-talk, how to identify and replace thinking errors, how to conquer (or master) worry, and detached mindfulness. She will learn the difference between realistic and unrealistic thinking, and that her fears are irrational and not an accurate predictor of what's to come. We also will discuss self-esteem, self-confidence, and the importance of being proactive, all of which will improve once your child begins to successfully face her fears. For the behavior part, you and your child will learn the Face Your Fears approach, which states that one must face his or her fears to overcome them. Thus, your child will learn that avoidance of anxiety-provoking situations is not the answer to dealing with fears. We also will work on understanding and eliminating nervous behaviors, such as reassurance seeking and asking an excessive amount of questions.

Figure 3 is an extension of Figure 2, with the treatment techniques for each part noted.

It is essential that parents are empathic and understanding during this process of treating the anxiety disorder. It is critical that parents do not blame, criticize, or tease their child for their anxiety disorder in any way, and that siblings are prevented from doing the same. Many parents interpret their child's anxiety-related behaviors as a product of oppositionality. However, this is rarely the case. The majority of the time, a child's seemingly oppositional behavior is a direct expression of his anxiety. It is important to conceptualize these behaviors as part of the anxiety disorder. For example, avoidance behaviors, resistance to change, and inflexibility all are common behaviors associated with a childhood anxiety disorder.

Finally, let me provide some guidance on how to make this book work best for you and your child. First of all, providing support, encouragement, and communicating confidence in your child and in his ability to face his fears is one of the greatest gifts you could give to your anxious child in his life. This is part of being an authoritative parent. As his parent, your child looks to you for signals and cues that he can charter into new territory and not be harmed. It is up to you to confirm this for him and emphasize that, not only will he not be harmed, but he will be helped and strengthened by taking what will feel like a huge risk. Think about the classic children's book *We're Going on a Bear Hunt* by Michael Rosen: "We can't go over it, we can't go under it. Oh no! We've got to go through it!" Basically, there is no other way but through. Of the children with anxiety disorders, those whose parents demonstrate that they fully believe in their child and his ability to master

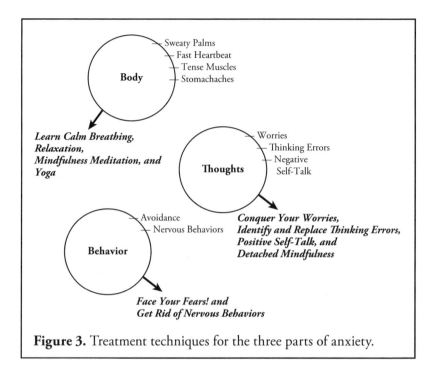

Figure 3. Treatment techniques for the three parts of anxiety.

the anxiety do the best in therapy and have the best outcomes. I also recommend using humor with your child, staying positive, and reminding your child to use the strategies and tools he learns from reading his book. Finally, I encourage you to talk to your child about the process that is involved in overcoming his anxieties. For example, making the following comments will help:

- ▶ (When doing relaxation): "You are practicing your calm breathing because you are going to use it when you begin to face your fears. You are doing a great job preparing yourself. I'm so proud of you!"
- ▶ (When doing self-talk note cards): "We are making these positive self-talk note cards to help you change the things you say to yourself when you are nervous. Using the note cards will help you feel better and calm."

▸ (When making hierarchy): "Together, we are making a list of all of the things that are hard to do because they make you feel nervous or scared. We are doing this because eventually you will face these fears, one step at a time. Remember that the book explains that you never will be forced to do these things. But I *will* encourage you to do them."

▸ (When facing their fears): "I know this is so hard for you, and that you feel nervous. But, remember what the book (or Dr. Zucker) says about this: You are not expected to like the nervous feeling, but you can handle it, it is not harmful to you. And, it will go away and it will get easier with practice. I am so proud of you and you should be very, very proud of yourself."

▸ (When refusing to provide reassurance, which may be one of the steps on their hierarchy): "I know this is hard for you, but we both know that I can't _____ (e.g., give you the answer you want to hear, tell you it will be OK, tell you what we're doing tomorrow, let you sleep in my bed, tell you who is going to be there). If I do _____ (same as first blank), it will make you feel better right now, but will make the overall anxiety much, much worse. Remember, you have to go through being nervous before it gets better. I know you can do it."

(Additional parental responses can be found in Chapter 12.)

It is always appropriate to answer your child's questions about the process and the purpose behind doing the activities that help her face her fears. However, if your child asks these questions repetitively, then it may be a symptom of anxiety (especially if asking a lot of questions is one of her reassurance-seeking behaviors). It will be important not to answer the questions over and over again. Instead, you can refer your child to her book to find the solutions.

Managing your own reaction to your child's anxiety and anxious behaviors is an important component of the treatment. Your child needs a strong foundation to help contain himself and his fears, and he will benefit from stability and a predictable reaction from you as he addresses his anxiety. Consistency in reading the chapters and doing the exercises is also very important, particularly for anxious children who are comforted by predictability. Many parents have told me that they use the strategies their child learns for their own benefit, and many practice relaxation and use calm breathing to manage their own anxiety. Because anxiety disorder tends to run in families, you may find that either you or someone else in your child's family also suffers from an anxiety disorder. If this is the case, it may be equally important to get your own treatment or treatment for other family members living in the home. Research shows that parental anxiety management (PAM), regardless of if there is parental anxiety or not, improves a child's outcome in the treatment of the child's anxiety, so it is also advisable for parents of anxious children to learn how to manage their own anxiety.

What About Professional Help and Medication?

Using this self-help program is an excellent first step in addressing the anxiety, and it is my goal and hope that this will be enough—that by the time you complete it, your child no longer will suffer from an anxiety disorder, and you and your family will be free from the limitations associated with it. Of course, you may be using this book in conjunction with ongoing psychotherapy, which can be very helpful. If you are using this as a form of self-help for your child, and at the completion of the program your child continues to have symptoms that cause an interference in his or her life, I recommend that you seek professional assistance. In this case, please refer to the last pages of this book for resources, or ask your child's pediatrician or school for a recommendation.

There are two main classes of medications used to treat anxiety in children and adults: *antidepressants* (which include SSRIs, or selective serotonin reuptake inhibitors; SNRIs, or serotonin norepinephrine reuptake inhibitors; TCAs, or tricyclic antidepressants; and "atypical" antidepressants) and *antianxiety medications* (which include benzodiazepines and buspirone). Both classes have been shown to decrease symptoms of anxiety and generally are considered to be safe. Antidepressants take a longer time to take effect, usually requiring 2–6 weeks before reaching a therapeutic level, and must be taken daily. Antianxiety medications take effect immediately and, in some cases, can be taken on an "as-needed" basis. In many cases, these medications will be prescribed in combination. Sometimes, an antipsychotic medication will be added to enhance the efficiency of the antidepressants or antianxiety medications. If prescribed, it usually is a very low dose and often will be discontinued once the child's symptoms improve. Psychiatrists and pediatricians (both of whom are medical doctors) are able to prescribe these medications. Table 1 lists commonly prescribed antidepressants, antianxiety medications, and the newer antipsychotics, as well as their common side effects.

It is very important to report all side effects to your child's doctor, although many of them will subside within a few weeks of your child being on the medication. In addition to the side effects listed, if your child has any of the following symptoms: shortness of breath, fainting, disorientation, intense muscle tension, or fever, then contact your doctor immediately, or take your child to the emergency room. Also, there are other rare side effects, so as a general rule if your child experiences any somatic complaints that are substantial, even if they are not in this list, let your doctor know.

It is good practice for a medical doctor to use a drug's side effects to the patient's advantage. For example, anxious children who have trouble sleeping or are underweight might be prescribed Remeron because it has the side effects of drowsiness and weight gain. It is important to note an SSRI's side effect of initial increased anxiety typically results from starting on a dose that is too high; in this case, lowering the dose should help. Wellbutrin should not be prescribed for individuals with eating disorders due to the risk

Table 1
Antianxiety Medications

Type	Brand (Generic) Name	Side Effects
Antidepressants		
SSRIs	Brintellix (vortioxetine) Celexa (citalopram) Lexapro (escitalopram) Luvox (fluvoxamine) Paxil (paroxetine) Prozac (fluoxetine) Viibryd (vilazodone) Zoloft (sertraline)	Common: low sex drive, delayed orgasm Occasional: stomachaches, diarrhea, tremor, initial increased anxiety, agitation, irritability, headaches, sedation, trouble sleeping
SNRIs	Cymbalta (duloxetine) Effexor (venlafaxine) Pristiq (desvenlafaxine)	Same as SSRIs
TCAs	Anafranil (clomipramine) Elavil (amitriptyline) Pamelor (nortriptyline) Tofranil (imipramine)	Dry mouth, constipation, dizziness, tremor, sedation, anxiety, weight gain, hypotension
Other	Desyrel (trazodone) Remeron (mirtazapine) Serzone (nefazodone) Wellbutrin (bupropion)	Desyrel (trazodone): drowsiness, priapsism (erection that will not go away) Remeron (mirtazapine): drowsiness, weight gain Serzone (nefazodone): drowsiness, irritability Wellbutrin (bupropion): irritability, insomnia, anxiety, dry mouth, weight loss, constipation

Type	Brand (Generic) Name	Side Effects
Antianxiety		
Benzodiazepines	Ativan (lorazepam) Klonopin (clonazepam) Valium (diazepam) Xanax (alprazolam)	Drowsiness, fatigue, lethargy, impaired coordination, memory problems, withdrawal symptoms
Beta Blockers	Inderal (propranolol) Tenormin (atenolol)	Lightheadedness, exercise intolerance
Other	Buspar (buspirone)	Dizziness
Atypical Antipsychotics/ Mood Stabilizers (often used to enhance effectiveness of antidepressants)	Abilify (aripiprazole)* Geodon (ziprasidone)*, ** Latuda (lurasidone)*,** Risperdal (risperidone) Saphris (asenapine) Seroquel (quetiapine) Zyprexa (olanzapine)	Common: increased appetite, weight gain, sedation, dizziness, dry mouth, blurred vision, muscle spasms, diabetes, restlessness, tremor Rare: tardive dyskinesia (repetitive, involuntary movements)

*do not have diabetes as a side effect
**do not cause increased appetite or weight gain

of seizures (sometimes children with anxiety, especially OCD, can have co-occurring eating disorders). Anytime a medication is stopped, it must be done in a gradual fashion. Suddenly stopping a medication can lead to significant side effects, particularly for Effexor and Paxil, which are known for withdrawal symptoms if they are discontinued abruptly. Finally, doctors should be informed of any other health problem or condition your child may have, as this may influence which type of drug is prescribed.

The research on anxiety disorders treatment has concluded that CBT or CBT in combination with medication is effective. Some studies have shown that CBT leads to better long-term results with lower incidence of relapse (Barlow, 2004; Hollon et al., 2006). The benefits of CBT appear to be longer lasting and continue even after therapy has been concluded; whereas medication benefits occur when the child is on the medication (see http://www.abct.org for more information). A recent study indicated that CBT for anxiety during childhood offered long-term protection from later suicidal ideation (Wolk et al., 2015).

A large NIMH-funded study conducted at Johns Hopkins University by Dr. John Walkup and colleagues (2008) examined almost 500 children with anxiety disorders and found that 80% improved from CBT plus SSRIs (they used up to 200mg of sertraline) whereas 60% improved from CBT alone (55% improved on sertraline alone). My caveat to these results (particularly given that my own results with working with children with anxiety disorders is much higher than 60%, or even, 80%) is that the researchers, for the purpose of interrater reliability and a sound research design, used a manualized treatment program for the CBT component (they used the excellent *Coping Cat Program* developed by Dr. Philip Kendall at Temple University), which generally differs from the actual course of CBT therapy a child will receive in the context of a meaningful relationship with a clinician in private practice. Basically, what I am saying is that the relationship I have with the children I work with, and the flexibility to structure therapy according to their own specific needs and ideal timeline, results in a better success rate, and this is from "just CBT" (no medication). I believe medication has its place and at times, I recommend it for children with whom I work (usually those with an OCD diagnosis), after we've not seen as much improvement as we would like after a certain period of time (and usually this pertains to the continuation of intrusive thoughts and images; the treatment of the avoidance behavior or compulsions is usually successful on its own).

Medication often leads to greater short-term benefit, but the effects are not as strong as CBT in the long run. When making the decision to have your child begin medication, consider my two rules of thumb: (1) Your child should only begin medication if, after 3 months of cognitive behavioral therapy, you, your child, and the therapist feel there has been little or no improvement; and (2) your child should *only* be on medication if he or she also continues to attend therapy with a licensed therapist. I believe there is one exception to the first rule of thumb: Your child may benefit from taking an immediate-acting benzodiazepine (e.g., Klonopin, Xanax) if there is an imminent situation that warrants it (e.g., your child has a fear of flying and will be flying in the very near future or your child refuses to go to school and is missing most days), and only during the situation (not to be used regularly). In addition, before medication is considered, you may want to look into testing for a gluten or dairy intolerance or allergy, or even trying a gluten and diary-free diet for 2–3 months, as there is increasingly good evidence that suggests that going gluten-free (or limiting it) can reduce anxiety (see Resources under Nutrition and Dietary). Other dietary modifications such as adopting a low- or no-sugar lifestyle and/or limiting processed foods may be worthwhile to try before considering medication, as these additives can stimulate a child's system and impact mood. If medication is used, once the child improves to the point at which the anxiety no longer meets the criteria for a disorder, and this progress is maintained for 6–12 months, he or she gradually can be taken off the medication, under the supervision of the prescribing doctor. The majority of the time, medication should not be considered a permanent treatment, but only a temporary one. Consult your doctor or a psychiatrist for more information.

In summary, anxiety disorders are the most common psychological disorder of childhood. CBT is the most effective and empirically supported treatment approach for anxiety disorders, and it views anxiety has having three components: body, thoughts, and behavior. We will address these three parts of anxiety, starting by identifying your child's anxiety-provoking situations and avoidance behaviors in the next chapter.

EXERCISE

Chapter 1 EXERCISE

Tips for Parents

1. As a reminder, exercises are to be completed by you and your child together. The exercises appear the same in your child's book, thus you'll note that the exercises in your book are written to your child.

2. When completing this exercise with your child, try to elicit as many personal examples as possible.

Fill in the Bubbles

Directions: You and your parent will do this together. In each of the bubbles, write in the three parts of anxiety. Next to each part (bubble), write your own examples of your experience with anxiety. For example, you can write down what specific things happen to your body when you are anxious.

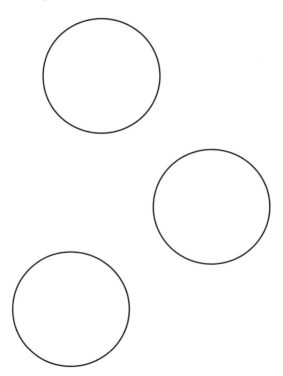

CHAPTER

2

Making Your Team and Team Goals

Kimberly and her parents learned that she has generalized anxiety disorder (GAD) and that she will need to learn how to relax her body, change the ways she thinks, and face her fears. She realized that there were a lot of things she avoided doing because they made her feel afraid or uncomfortable. Kimberly and her mom worked together to make a list of all of the situations that cause Kimberly to feel anxious or worried. They made the list into a ladder, so Kimberly could see the different steps she would take to overcome her anxiety, and note her progress along the way. Kimberly decided that her first step would be to reduce the number of times she checked on her dog to only twice a day.

In this chapter, your child will learn the following:
1. the "Face Your Fears" philosophy,
2. a case example of Thelma, who overcame her separation anxiety by facing her fears, and
3. how to form a team and make a ladder (hierarchy) for achieving goals.

These topics will be addressed in this chapter, and the exercise that you will complete with your child after you each read Chapter 2 of your respective books will be discussed. This chapter also will include a section on the importance of not providing reassurance.

This is a shorter chapter to read, but the exercise that you and your child will complete is longer than most of the other exercises in this book. The exercise (Making Your Team and Team Goals) is going to be fun and will set the stage for your child's treatment goals: facing his or her fears. It is through facing his own fears that your child will learn to overcome them and break free from the cycle of anxiety. When your child avoids situations that evoke anxiety, this is called *avoidance behavior* because she is avoiding something in reaction to the anxiety (in acceptance and commitment therapy, it's called *experiential avoidance,* which is where the goal of tolerating the unpleasant emotions and sensations come in). Think about it; it makes sense. Your child's mentality is akin to:

> When I _____ (separate from Mom, raise my hand in class, go near a dog), I feel completely scared, threatened, nervous, and/or terrified, so of course I don't want to do it again.

However, each time that your child avoids something because it makes her feel anxious, *the anxiety wins* and becomes reinforced and strengthened, and *your child loses.* But each time your child does something that makes her feel anxious, *she wins* and *the anxiety loses.* It is your child against the anxiety (in the kids' companion book I call this, "You vs. Anxiety"), and it is certain that as your child faces her fears, she *will* win!

Although you learned a little about Thelma in the last chapter, the following is directly from your child's book and gives more detail about Thelma's experience, as well as her process of facing her fears:

> Eight-year-old Thelma was one of the children I worked with in therapy. She was very nice, very smart, and very nervous about being separated from her mom. If her mom went out in the front of the house to take out the trash, Thelma would become anxious—her heart would beat fast, and she would stop doing whatever she was doing to go

to the window and watch her mom. Thelma would worry that something bad would happen to her and that she wouldn't come back. Thelma also did not like to be in a different room than her mom, and when her mom would go in another room, Thelma would ask her to sing a song so Thelma would always know where she was. She refused to sleep in her own bed at night even though her mom would try to get her to sleep alone, but Thelma would cry and cry and beg her mom to be able to sleep with her. Sometimes, Thelma's mom needed to go out without her and a babysitter would come over; this upset Thelma so much that she would get sick and throw up. As soon as her mom would come home, Thelma would feel better. This made it very hard for her mom to leave the house without her!

Thelma had separation anxiety, which meant that she got very nervous and worried when she was separated from her mom and worried about bad things happening to her mom. She did her best to *avoid* being separated from her, because this was the thing that made her feel so scared. Each time Thelma was clinging onto her mother and *avoided* being separated from her, *the anxiety would win and she would lose.* Even though staying near her mother helped her to feel better at the time, it actually made the anxiety much worse overall. Thelma learned that she had to face her fears to overcome them. How did she do it?

Thelma and her team (her mom, sister, and me, Dr. Zucker) worked together to make a list of all of the things that felt scary to her and that were hard to do. Then, Thelma and I put the list in order, from easiest to hardest, and wrote them all on a poster board, in the form of a ladder. Each step on the ladder was one of the things that was hard for her to do. Thelma learned how to relax and take deep breaths, learned that her fears were not realistic (it was perfectly safe for her mom to take out the trash), and learned what to say to herself to help herself deal with the scary thoughts and feelings. Thelma also learned that she was making thinking mistakes and worked on correcting them. Finally, she understood that she needed to face her fears, one step (or fear) at a time. She knew that when she was facing her fears, she would have to handle feeling some anxiety, but that the anxiety would go away with time and practice. Most importantly, Thelma was told that she would not have to take any of the steps until she was ready; Thelma would not be forced to face her fears. Instead, Thelma would be *encouraged* by her team to face her fear—she would be cheered on.

Thelma named her ladder "Climbing to Confidence" because she felt that her separation anxiety made her feel less confident about herself. By facing her fears, she would feel more confident. This is what Thelma's ladder looked like:

Climbing to Confidence

(top)	Mom goes out of town without you.
	Go on a sleepover at a friend's house.
	Mom goes out for the day without you.
	Go on a play date at a friend's house.
	Mom goes out for 1 hour, then 2 hours without you.
	Mom goes out for 15 minutes, then 30 minutes without you.
	Sleep in your bed alone one night this week (then 2, 4, 5, and 7 nights).
	You use a public bathroom on your own (without Mom).
	Mom takes the trash out and you stay focused on the TV.
	Mom stays upstairs while you stay downstairs (for 5, 10, 15, and 30 minutes, then for 1 hour).

(bottom)	Mom goes into other rooms without singing to you. You stay in living room while Mom is in kitchen (for 5, 10, 15, 20, and 30 minutes).

Thelma practiced her relaxation and deep breathing, read her self-talk note cards, studied the thinking mistakes that she made and how to think more correct or realistic thoughts, and used her tools to master her worry. When she was ready, Thelma took the first step on her ladder: to go in the living room while her mom was in the nearby kitchen. She started slow, doing it for 5 minutes, then did it for longer periods of time—10, 15, 20, and 30 minutes—eventually being able to be in the living room alone for more than an hour! It wasn't easy, but it wasn't nearly as hard as she thought it would be. The first time she did it, she called to her mom, who popped her head in the living room and told Thelma that she was facing her fears and doing a fantastic job. She did it again and again, and then it became very easy, and did not cause her to feel scared or nervous at all. By the third time, she did not have to ask her mom to come in, and she learned to feel comfortable being in the living room alone. She was able to relax and enjoy watching TV and reading a book. Then Thelma felt ready to take the second step: her mother would go into other rooms in the house while Thelma was in the living room or her bedroom, but her mom would not sing to her. Again, she felt nervous and scared the first time they practiced, but it got easier and easier with each practice, and soon Thelma did not feel nervous when her mother left the room. Thelma remembered to do her breathing and read her self-talk note cards. She also told herself that feeling nervous was normal, but that it would get better, and it did.

Your child is told that like Thelma, she will build a ladder and team to help her face her fears. Looking at Thelma's ladder will help your child do this.

To be part of your child's team, you'll have to identify what you need to do to make the steps on the ladder go smoothly. As described above, Thelma's mom did many things to help Thelma to not feel anxious, including:

- ▶ singing to Thelma as she went in different rooms in the house,
- ▶ allowing Thelma to sleep with her in her bed, and
- ▶ avoiding leaving the house without her as much as possible.

These behaviors served to *accommodate* Thelma's anxiety. Unfortunately, such behaviors tend to make anxiety worse. Loving, caring, warm parents want to put their child at ease and make the anxiety lessen. Loving, caring, warm parents end up *unintentionally reinforcing* the anxiety by accommodating it and by providing their child with reassurance. It gives the child the message that her anxiety *is* that bad—it's so bad that it's worth addressing and focusing on and even changing the way we live. You know better than anyone what it's like for your child to turn to you to make everything OK. This may come out in the form of questions, such as, "What will we be doing tomorrow?" and "Will you definitely be home in an hour?" and "You still love me, right?" or it may come out in behavior, such as when your child throws a tantrum if he or she isn't allowed to sleep in bed with you. In an effort to soothe your child and make it better, you give into these demands—you answer the questions, you avoid doing things that are hard for your child to handle. The most wonderful parents do this instinctively. The funny thing is, it doesn't work! It provides temporary relief at best. Your child likely asks these questions repetitively, but the answers do not solve the worry or lessen the anxiety. Rather, the answers give the anxiety credibility.

You are the instrumental part of your child's team in facing his fears. As such an important team member, it is essential that your role entail being supportive and encouraging, but *not* accommodating. For example, Thelma's mother needed to learn that she had to stop singing as she went in different rooms, could not allow Thelma to sleep with her (nor sleep with Thelma in Thelma's room), and could not stay at home to avoid prompting a meltdown. Her mother stopped giving these accommodations in a gradual way so as not to overwhelm Thelma. Once Thelma endorsed that she was ready to face her fears, her mom would meet her at that goal. For instance, once Thelma felt ready to have her mother leave the room without singing to her, Thelma's mother had to stop singing, even if during the exposure, Thelma got upset or requested that her mom sing.

In sum, you will stop accommodating your child's anxiety in a step-by-step fashion, as she takes the steps on her ladder, but you will need to be firm and consistent by not giving in. Instead of accommodating, you will cue her to use her strategies to manage the anxiety. At times it will be quite challenging and possibly very upsetting to you; however, it is necessary to end these accommodations in order for your child to become anxiety-free. Don't forget that one of the ways that you can help your child deal with not having you accommodate his anxiety is to comment on the process: "I know this is hard for you, and it's hard for me, too. A part of me wants to sing to you because I know it will make you feel better in that moment, but it will make the anxiety worse overall. It will make the anxiety bigger and stronger, and as a team, we need to fight it by not giving in. It will get easier with practice." Also, remind your child to use his tools by saying, "What can you do right now to help yourself feel better?" If he does not know, remind him of the strategies he can use: breathing, self-talk, conquer worry strategies, and so on.

The exercise for this chapter involves creating your child's team and the ladder (the hierarchy of anxiety-provoking situations). I deliberately placed the exercise of creating the hierarchy as one of the earliest projects because it frames the goals that your child is working toward. Below are two additional sample ladders and brief descriptions of the exposure process. Reviewing these will help you better understand the process of making the ladder and ordering the steps from least to most anxiety-producing.

Sample 1: James (Snake Phobia)

Taking Steps With Snakes

(top)	Be near a live snake out of its cage up close (within 6 inches).
	Be near a live snake out of its cage from a distance (2 feet away).
	Be near a live snake in its cage up close (within 6 inches).
	Be near a live snake in its cage from a distance (2 feet away).
	Touch a snakeskin.
	Standing near a bush (and when it is rustled by an animal).
	Watching a video with snakes.
	Hearing the sounds of a snake (hissing sound).
	Looking at pictures of snakes.
	Reading about snakes.
(bottom)	Talking about snakes.

James and I made his ladder together and he was very involved in planning the exposures. For example, he went to the library and checked out books on snakes and movies with snake scenes. We watched a scene from *The Black Stallion* in which the boy in the movie had a terrifying encounter with a cobra snake, watched an informational video on how to care for your pet snake (not that James's goals included having a pet snake!), and watched the scene from the *Harry Potter* movie that included an animated snake. When it came time to be near live snakes, James and I started with a trip to the National Zoo's Reptile House. At first, he kept his distance, but on our second visit, he felt comfortable enough to go close up to the glass enclosure. We went to the pet store three times together, and each time he got closer and closer to the live snake (we requested that the snake be taken out of the cage). James and I laughed about the fact that the same employee helped us every time, but had no idea what we were doing there. We could tell by the third visit that she thought it was a little strange that we wanted to see the snake, but not too close, and certainly did not want to touch or hold it (of course, the assumption in a pet store is that we would be interested in buying a snake). I told James that it's our right to go into the pet store, without buying (or even handling) the pet snakes! After our last trip to the pet store, I took James to an ice cream shop for an ice cream treat. He enjoyed this reward immensely (mainly the celebration and acknowledgement of his progress and success) and felt proud of himself for all of his hard work on facing his fears. Eventually, he visited the house of his friend with the pet snake. James attended a total of 12 sessions of CBT with me, and by the end, he no longer met the criteria for a snake phobia. His parents commented that James seemed happier and more confident in himself.

Sample 2: Ruth (OCD)

Getting Over Germs!

(top)	Using a public bathroom and rewearing your clothes the next day.
	Using a public bathroom and washing your clothes only once afterward.

	Touching the door on the way out of the public bathroom with your hands.
	Touching the faucet in a public bathroom with your hands.
	Touching the stall door lock and handle of a public bathroom with your hands.
	Flushing the toilet in a public bathroom using your hands.
	Using a public bathroom and touching the door on the way in with your hands.
	Using a public bathroom.
	Eating from the school cafeteria.
	Eating homemade cookies and brownies.
	Eating from a "shared" bowl in a public place.
	Eating from a "shared" bowl at a party.
(bottom)	Eating at home with an "unclean" utensil (hand-washed only).

Ruth's treatment involved a lot of education. First of all, she needed to understand that germs are neither dangerous nor threatening. She learned that we are exposed to germs every day and that we need germs to be healthy (I explained, in detail, that our bodies make special things called *antibodies* that prevent us from getting sick and that the only way our bodies can make these special antibodies is to be exposed to germs). Ruth also learned that germs are all over everything, a part of our environment, and that we cannot see germs. I emphasized that I was not trying to make her more anxious; rather, I was helping her understand that germs are a normal part of life. I explained the difference between being hygienic (washing our hands after using the bathroom and before and after meals, washing our clothes) and being irrational (refusing to eat from a bowl of chips at a party, washing clothes three times in between wears). I assured her that taking the steps on her ladder would not make her sick, and I modeled these steps for her. In one session, I literally took some chips and put them on the floor, then picked them up and ate them. She looked disgusted with me as I did this, but I told her I was doing something extreme to show her that nothing bad would happen. I reassured her the next week that I did not get sick from eating the chips, and in fact, they tasted just as good as if I'd eaten them from the bag. I also assured her that while I do not make it a habit of eating off of the floor, I'm not afraid of doing it.

Facing one's fear is at the core of cognitive-behavioral treatment for anxiety disorders. Up until now, your child has likely been accommodating her anxiety, living her life avoiding those situations that cause her to feel nervous, uncomfortable, and scared. As her parent, you have no doubt joined her in living this way. By forming a "team" and developing "team goals," you are helping your child begin to take back control in her life and to overcome her anxiety and fears. The next chapter will focus on learning how to relax and calm the body.

Chapter 2 EXERCISE

EXERCISE (vertical, left margin)

Tips for Parents

1. Because forming the hierarchy involves listing many or all of your child's fear situations, he may feel a little over-whelmed (or anxious) about the prospect of having to complete the situations on his ladder. This is why it is crucial for you to remind your child of two things:

   a. Your child will not have to face his fears just yet; first, he will learn many tools and strategies to manage the task of facing fears.

   b. Your child will not be forced to face his fears. Rather, your child will go at his own pace. Although you will encourage your child, you will not force him to face his fears.

2. When developing the list of anxiety-provoking situations for your child, you may want to ask yourself the following questions: What things are hard for your child to do because he is anxious about doing them? What things do you avoid doing because they are upsetting/anxiety-provoking to your child? What are other children you know capable of doing that your child is not (e.g., riding a bike, going on a play date)? You also may want to ask extended family members or your closest friends what they observe to be challenging for your child to do because of his anxiety and include these situations in the ladder.

3. Remember to be very encouraging with your child as the two of you complete the ladder. You want to make it as positive and fun as possible, and ensure that it is not a shaming experience for him. Some children are sensitive about listing the many different things that are hard for them to do. If your child begins to feel this way, or expresses

embarrassment about his anxiety, then remind him of how common it is: that many children have anxiety. Tell him, "It's the most common problem for kids, and at least 1 out of every 8 children have problems with anxiety" and "She wrote this book for a reason—there are a lot of kids with anxiety out there." It is essential that you do not allow his embarrassment to prevent you from doing the exercise; is it possible that your child may be magnifying the embarrassment as a way to avoid facing his fears. In this case, label it as resistance and talk with your child (in a calm, nonblaming tone) about his concerns about treating the anxiety. Also, tell him how proud you are of him; provide positive reinforcement like praise and reward ("Let's do this and then watch your favorite movie"). If needed, you can bring up the importance of being proactive and discuss living by our values, as discussed in Chapter 12.

4. As recommended below, I always leave a few spaces between some of the steps just in case you and your child decide to add some more situations (this often occurs once you have begun the exposure process).

5. When doing the exposures on their ladder, children will find it helpful if you can model for them first. So, if your child has social anxiety and she worries about sending food back in a restaurant or spilling something in public, show her it's not so bad by first doing it yourself. This also will help her feel more confident about being able to do the exposures.

6. Finally, it is ideal if you can make the ladder as specific as possible, including the duration of the exposure, starting out small and gradually making it longer. For example, Thelma started out with her mom in the kitchen while she was in the living room alone for 5 minutes and gradually made it up to 30 minutes. It's also best to use positive lan-

guage like "stand near a bush" instead of "don't run away from the bush."

Making Your Team and Team Goals

Who Is on Your Team? Write in the names of the members of your team in the blanks below. You do not have to fill in all of the blanks. Your team will be at least three people: You (the captain), whoever is reading the parent book (usually Mom or Dad), and me (Dr. Zucker). Other people you can include on your team are your grandparents, sister or brother, babysitter or nanny, pets, and your therapist if you have one. Your team members all will help you to face your fears in different ways. For example, Thelma's dog, Sniffy, was on her team and Sniffy helped her face her fears by being with her in the beginning when she was nervous about her mom leaving her alone in the living room. Sniffy also gave her extra licks when she was happy about doing such a great job in facing her fears.

Your Team:

1. Team Captain: _____
                                 (your name here)
2. _____
3. _____
4. _____
5. _____
6. _____

Team Goals: Making Your Ladder

You will need the following materials to make your ladder:

- ▸ Blank note cards
- ▸ Poster board (white or another light color)
- ▸ Markers
- ▸ Pen or pencil
- ▸ Stickers (stars, happy faces, whatever you want)

EXERCISE

To Make Your Ladder:

1. Using note cards and a pen or pencil, write down all of the different things that are hard for you to do or that you avoid doing because of anxiety and worry. Your parent will help you make this list. Write each of these things on a different note card (sometimes kids and their parents choose to write it down on a piece of paper before they write it on the note cards; either way works, just as long as each thing is written on a note card).

2. Use the floor or a table and spread out all of the note cards. Then look carefully at each of the note cards and put them in order from easiest to hardest (your parent will help). The easiest ones will be on the bottom and the hardest ones will be up at the top. Here is what Thelma's note cards looked like before she made them into a ladder:

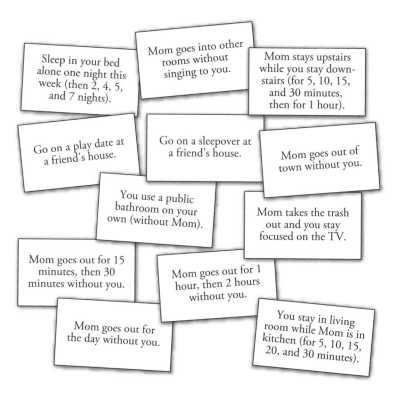

Sleep in your bed alone one night this week (then 2, 4, 5, and 7 nights).

Mom goes into other rooms without singing to you.

Mom stays upstairs while you stay downstairs (for 5, 10, 15, and 30 minutes, then for 1 hour).

Go on a play date at a friend's house.

Go on a sleepover at a friend's house.

Mom goes out of town without you.

You use a public bathroom on your own (without Mom).

Mom takes the trash out and you stay focused on the TV.

Mom goes out for 15 minutes, then 30 minutes without you.

Mom goes out for 1 hour, then 2 hours without you.

Mom goes out for the day without you.

You stay in living room while Mom is in kitchen (for 5, 10, 15, 20, and 30 minutes).

EXERCISE

3. Now count your note cards. How many do you have?

_____

4. Come up with a title for your ladder. Write the name here:

_____

Now, write the title at the top of the poster board.

5. Use the poster board and markers to draw a great big lad-
    der with steps, under where you wrote the title. The num-
    ber of steps you draw should be the same as the number of
    note cards you have. Leave a little space here and there in
    between some of the steps, just in case you decide to add
    more things later on.
6. Write the steps, from easiest to hardest, on the ladder using
    the markers.

The stickers will be used once you start doing the steps. We
won't begin doing this just yet; first you need to learn some tools
(or ways) to deal with your anxious feelings and worries. You will
first learn how to help the **body** part of anxiety. In the next chapter,
you will learn about relaxation and deep breathing.

CHAPTER

3

Relaxing the Body

Kimberly started to notice that when she was anxious or worried, her body felt different. Her muscles were tight and tense, her heartbeat would speed up, and she seemed to always have a stomachache or a headache. Kimberly and her mom learned different ways to relax her body, and she started to learn how to loosen her muscles and slow her heartbeat down. Kimberly also liked practicing relaxing imagery with her dad before he tucked her in at night.

THIS chapter focuses on addressing the physiological or body part of anxiety. In Chapter 1, you and your child learned that the body has a reaction when you feel anxious. In this chapter, you and your child will learn how to do the five types of relaxation:

1. calm breathing,
2. progressive muscle relaxation (PMR),
3. relaxing imagery,
4. mindfulness meditation, and
5. yoga.

Learning how to relax should be a positive experience for your child, so try to frame it that way when the two of you complete the exercise at the end. The goal is for your child to become a master of relaxation. Because it is physiologically impossible to be relaxed and anxious at the same time, if your child uses his relaxation skills at the time he feels anxious, it will help alleviate the anxiety. In recent years, many helpful (and typically free) apps have been developed to teach and help practice relaxation (I have listed some of my favorite ones in the Resources for Parents section at the end of the parent book, although new ones are constantly arising). I, along with my colleague, Dr. Mary Alvord, and her son, Bryce Alvord, recorded a CD entitled, *Relaxation and Self-Regulation Techniques for Children and Teens.* Given how many of the children or parents I work with have access to iTunes or MP3 players, they often download a few of the recordings. You can substitute the scripts below with one of the apps or CD tracks, or offer them all to your child to see which she prefers.

The following sections include scripts for you to use with your child to help her relax.

Calm Breathing

When breathing in a calm, relaxed way, you breathe in through your nose and out through your mouth. As you breathe in through your nose, allow the air to travel all the way down to your lower belly. This is the opposite from breathing in an anxious, tense way when your breathing is shallow and the air only goes down as far as the upper part of your chest.

Have your child try doing this: *Breathe in through your nose for the count of 4 and then out through your mouth for the count of 4.* As she does this, have her try to get the air that she breathes in to go all the way to the bottom of her belly, below her belly button. It helps to have her put her hands on this part of her abdomen and then try to get her hands to move up and down as she breathes in and out. Encourage her to try not to let any air stop, or get stuck, in the top of her chest; tell her to just let the air go in easily through her nose all of the way to the bottom of her belly. For younger children, you can help them learn by saying, "smell the roses and blow out the candles. There is a big bouquet of flowers—smell them all—and now there is a big birthday cake with lots and lots of candles—blow them all out . . . keep blowing . . . keep blowing."

Look at Thelma as she learns how to do calm breathing. Notice how her lower belly goes out as she breathes in.

Say the following to your child: *"Breathe in through your nose for the count of 4, hold the breath for a few seconds, and then slowly breathe out through your mouth for the count of 4."* To teach this, I demonstrate by lying on my back on the floor with a cork yoga block (you can use a book instead) placed on my upper chest. I show them how the block (resting on my upper chest) moves up and down when I am anxious, as I am only allowing the air to travel into my upper chest (the "shallow end"). Then I demonstrate what calm breathing looks like: The block continues to be on my upper chest, but this time, it remains still as the air slowly travels all the way down to my lower abdomen ("the deep end"), causing it to rise and fall with each incoming and outgoing breath. Once I show them how it's done, it's their turn to lie down with the block and practice both ways of breathing.

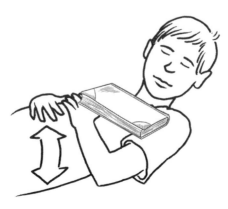

Sometimes kids will have a hard time catching their breath when they are anxious. If this happens, have your child try breathing in and out through only one nostril. Say the following to your child: *"Let's practice one-nostril breathing. Hold one of your nostrils closed and close your mouth, then breathe in and out through only one nostril."* It will help if the two of you practice together; this way you can model the pacing for her, showing her how to take long, slow breaths in and out through only one nostril. Start with the count of 5 (5 in and 5 out), gradually building up to the count of 10 (10 in and 10 out); I usually hold up my hand and count on my fingers as I practice with the child.

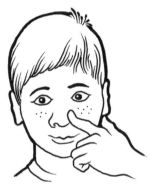

The most important thing to remember is that these breathing techniques must first be mastered when your child is calm.

Progressive Muscle Relaxation (PMR)

PMR is a type of relaxation that involves making your muscles relax by first tightening them up and holding them for the count of 5–10 seconds. Your child will do one section of the body at a time, starting with his hands and going all the way down to his feet. When your child does PMR, try to have him focus on what it feels like when his muscles are tight and tense and when they are loose and relaxed. Here is a script for you and your child to use to practice PMR:

1. Start by making tight fists with your hands, imagining that you are squeezing the juice out of a lemon. Hold your fists nice and tight and count to 10. Then let go and shake it out (shake your hands out). Notice how it feels when your muscles are tight and tense versus when they are loose and relaxed.

2. Now pull your arms into your body next to your ribs. Tighten up your bicep and forearms muscles, but do not make fists or tighten your hands. Hold it for 1, 2, 3, 4, 5, 6, 7, 8, 9, and 10, then let it go and shake it out. Remember to notice what your muscles feel like when they are tense and when they are loose. Sometimes once you loosen them, your muscles will feel a little tingly.

3. Bring your shoulders all the way up toward your ears and tighten them up; this also should make the back of your neck tight. Hold it for the count of 10, then allow your shoulders to drop down toward your hips. As you do this, say the word *relax* to yourself, and also breathe out slowly through your mouth.

4. Now pull your shoulders back and arch your back in toward your chest, trying to get your elbows to touch. Imagine that there is a string connected to your chest and someone is pulling the string up, lifting your chest up toward the ceiling. This will tighten your back. Hold it for 10 then let it go and feel the difference between tension and relaxation.

5. Squeeze and pull your stomach, or abdominal, muscles in toward your spine. Keep it tight for 10 seconds, then let it go.

6. Now squeeze your buttocks muscles (they are important, too!) and hold for 10 seconds, then let go and loosen them up.

7. Stick your legs and feet straight out in front of you and point your toes in toward your chest. This will tighten the muscles in your legs and thighs. Make the muscles as tight as you can and hold for 10 seconds, then let go and allow your legs to gently drop to the ground and relax.

8. Stick your legs and feet straight out in front of you again, but this time point your toes straight out away from you and tighten up the muscles in your legs, thighs, and feet. Try to get it so you feel a little cramping in the bottom of your feet. Hold for 10 seconds, then let go, allowing your legs to gently drop to the floor.

9. Now we will tighten up all of the muscles in your face. Start by clenching your teeth and jaw. Then squish up your nose, lifting it up, and close your eyes and squeeze the muscles around them, and tighten up your forehead. Hold this tightness in your whole face for 10 seconds, then let go and relax. Open your mouth a little bit and move your jaw from left to right and then in circles. This will allow the jaw to become even more relaxed.

10. Last step: WHOLE BODY! You want to go from being a stiff, tight robot to being a loose, relaxed rag doll! Start with tight fists, then add arms, bring shoulders up to your ears and then pull them back to tighten your back, squeeze your stomach into your spine, tighten your buttocks, put your legs out in front of you with your toes pointing out away from you and cramp up your feet, and tighten your jaw and whole face. HOLD FOR 10 SECONDS (ROBOT) and then LET GO (RAG DOLL), loosening every muscle in your body. I could tell if you were a really relaxed rag doll if I tried to lift up your arm and it felt very heavy and loose.

Relaxing Imagery

Relaxing imagery offers another type of relaxation, and it is best to first learn and practice it at home or in your therapist's office. This type of relaxation allows your child the opportunity to become deeply relaxed and really "let go" of tension and stress. You will guide your child in a guided relaxation as part of the exercise at the end of this chapter.

When preparing to practice, encourage your child to find a comfortable place to sit or lie down. Some kids really like to use pillows, too. If she wants to use pillows to get more comfortable, have her try putting one under her head, another one under her knees, and maybe one under each of her arms. You and your child may enjoy listening to some relaxing music (with no words) in the background. Here is a script for you to use with your child to teach her about relaxing imagery.

Once you are comfortable, I want you to close your eyes and take a deep breath in through your nose and out through your mouth. As you breathe in, imagine that you are breathing in clean, relaxing air and as you breathe out, let go of any stress or tension that you are holding onto. Breathing in, you let calm air go all the way down to the bottom of your belly. Breathing out, you let go of the air and your belly becomes flat. With each breath, you feel more and more relaxed.

Imagine that you are standing in a hallway. This is the most beautiful hallway you have ever been in—the floor is cushiony and soft, and the colors that surround you are all of your favorites. The temperature is perfect—cool but not too cool—and you feel a slight breeze on your face. You notice that your body begins to loosen up.

You begin to walk down the hallway, and as you do, you feel lighter and lighter. The hallway curves around to the left and then curves around to the right. As you are walking, you see that it is getting brighter and brighter, and then the hallway ends in a beautiful room.

This room is filled with windows, several of which are cracked open just a bit, allowing a nice, cool, refreshing breeze to flow through the room. Sunlight is streaming in through the windows. You walk into the room and there is a big, soft, fluffy couch up against the wall. You decide to sit and then lie down on the couch. Your body is completely supported by the couch and there is a large, fluffy pillow under your head, and another one under your knees, taking away any tension from your neck and shoulders and back and feet.

As you lie there you feel the sunlight on your body, covering you from head to toe, warming you, and you feel the cool breeze flowing over you. The combination of the warm sun and the cool breeze makes you feel even more relaxed, and you begin to fall into a deep state of relaxation. You remind yourself this is your time for relaxation. You have nowhere to go and nothing to do. Any thoughts that come into your mind simply flow in and flow out. You don't need to hold onto any thoughts—just let them flow by.

Just outside this room, there are some orange and grapefruit trees. This is a very safe, very relaxing place. Just past the trees is a beach. You begin to think about this beach and the ocean. You imagine yourself standing at the shoreline and can feel the wet sand as it goes in between your toes. You look out into the crystal clear water and see that there are the most beautiful fish swimming by. You look at the fish—they are all different colors—purple, turquoise, yellow, and black, and then you see a few starfish on the ocean floor. Then some beautiful stingrays swim by—

you like to watch as the water changes the shape of their bodies. You are very relaxed as you watch these fish.

Then you focus on the waves, and watch as they come into the shore and then go out back into the ocean. Flowing in and then flowing out and then just flowing along. Nature is very peaceful.

Lying back on the couch, you think more about these waves. In just a moment, you will imagine a wave coming over your body, and as it does, it will soothe and comfort you, and then it will slowly leave your body, taking away any remaining tension and tightness. The wave can be any color—blue, green, purple—or it can be clear. Imagine the wave slowly going over your toes, feet, and ankles. Then it goes up your legs, knees, and thighs. It goes over your hips, hands, arms, and stomach, all the way up to your shoulders, but not over your neck. The wave is warm and comforting. It hangs out for just a minute, relaxing and soothing all of your muscles. Then the wave begins to leave, taking away all remaining tension, going down your stomach, arms, hands, and hips, all the way down past your thighs, knees, legs, and ankles, and then finally leaves your feet and toes. You are now even more relaxed.

Take a moment to enjoy this relaxation, noticing how calm and slow your breathing is. In just a minute, count to 10, and imagine yourself climbing up a set of stairs. With each step, you become more and more alert, but still very relaxed. At the top of the stairs, there will be an archway. You will walk through the archway and then you will be back in your own room, taking with you all the feelings of relaxation.

One, take the first step.
Two, take the second step.
Three, take the third step.
Four, take the fourth step.
Five, take the fifth step.
Six, take the sixth step.
Seven, take the seventh step.
Eight, take the eighth step.
Nine, take the ninth step.
And ten, take the tenth step.

Walk through the archway, and you are back in your room. Remind yourself that you can become this relaxed anytime you'd like, and it will only take 5 minutes!

You and your child can practice relaxing imagery with this scene or with any other relaxing scene. Below are a few additional scenes that are not included in your child's book. You can use these scenes when helping your child practice relaxing imagery. When reading the scene, try to use a calm and soft voice; you may choose to play background music (without words) on a low volume. Your child also is encouraged to come up with his own mental picture of a relaxing scene, which can be a real or an imaginary place.

Alternative Scene #1: Forest Scene

This scene begins the same as the scene above, but involves going to the forest, rather than the beach.

Once you are comfortable, I want you to close your eyes and take a deep breath in through your nose and out through your mouth. As you breathe in, imagine that you are breathing in clean, relaxing air, and as you breathe out, let go of any stress or tension that you are holding onto. Breathing in, you let calm air go all the way down to the bottom of your belly. Breathing out, you let go of the air and your belly becomes flat. With each breath, you feel more and more relaxed.

Imagine that you are standing in a hallway. This is the most beautiful hallway you have ever been in—the floor is cushiony and soft, and the colors that surround you are all of your favorites. The temperature is perfect—cool but not too cool—and you feel a slight breeze on your face. You notice that your body begins to loosen up.

You begin to walk down the hallway and as you do, you feel lighter and lighter. The hallway curves around to the left and then curves around to the right. As you are walking, you see that it is getting brighter and brighter, and then the hallway ends in a magical forest. This forest is the most beautiful and serene place you have ever been. The floor on which you stand is soft, and as you take a few steps, you hear the crackling sound of the leaves that you step on. On the forest floor, there are spots of sunlight, and this creates a warm feeling inside of you. There is a slight breeze and you can smell the pine in the air. As you gently walk through the forest, you see a stream ahead and you decide to go near it.

You let your fingers gently touch the water as it glides over the rocks in the stream. Just down the stream are two deer drinking from its cool water. You notice that your body feels calm and light, and you are free from any thoughts. You are just focused on being in the forest and feeling very, very relaxed.

You continue to walk in the forest and see a soft patch of green grass. You decide to sit and then lie down on the green grass. Lying on your back, you look up at the sky again and see the tops of the trees sway from left to right and right to left. The wind is blowing the leaves and branches around, and you love to hear the sound of the wind as it blows. Feeling so calm and so relaxed, you decide to gently close your eyes. You continue to hear the sounds of the forest and feel the warmth of the sun and the coolness of the slight breeze. You are very, very relaxed and very safe. Take some time to enjoy this relaxed feeling. If you notice any part of your body that feels tight, just imagine that part loosening up, and tell the muscle to "let go." Notice how calm and slow your breathing is.

In just a minute, I will count to 10, and I want you to imagine yourself climbing up a set of stairs. With each step, you become more and more alert, but still very relaxed. At the top of the stairs, there will be an archway. You will walk through the archway, and then you will be back in your own room, taking with you all the feelings of relaxation.

One, take the first step.
Two, take the second step.
Three, take the third step.
Four, take the fourth step.
Five, take the fifth step.
Six, take the sixth step.
Seven, take the seventh step.
Eight, take the eighth step.
Nine, take the ninth step.
And ten, take the tenth step.

Walk through the archway and gently open your eyes. You are back in your own room. Remind yourself that you can become this relaxed anytime you'd like, and it will only take 5 minutes!

Alternative Scene #2: Raft Scene

This scene can either be used in lieu of the relaxation scene in your child's book, or in addition to it (when he is standing at the beach, before he returns to lying on the couch). If you are using it in lieu of the one in his book, it will begin the same way.

Once you are comfortable, I want you to close your eyes and take a deep breath in through your nose and out through your mouth. As you breathe in, imagine that you are breathing in clean, relaxing air and as you breathe out, let go of any stress or tension that you are holding onto. Breathing in, you let calm air go all the way down to the bottom of your belly. Breathing out, you let go of the air and your belly becomes flat. With each breath, you feel more and more relaxed.

Imagine that you are standing in a hallway. This is the most beautiful hallway you have ever been in—the floor is cushiony and soft, and the colors that surround you are all of your favorites. The temperature is perfect—cool but not too cool—and you feel a slight breeze on your face. You notice that your body begins to loosen up.

You begin to walk down the hallway, and as you do, you feel lighter and lighter. The hallway curves around to the left and then curves around to the right. As you are walking, you see that it is getting brighter and brighter, and then the hallway ends in a beautiful beach. This is the most beautiful beach you have ever seen. The sand is perfectly white and soft, and not too hot. The water is crystal clear and perfectly turquoise in color. You walk toward the shoreline and look out into the ocean. You can smell the salt in the air and hear the sound of the water as it gently hits the land. There are very few waves; the water is very calm. In front of you is a big, fully inflated raft. This raft is very special because it has a secret window on the bottom of it that lets you clearly see what's in the ocean. You decide to give the raft a push into the water and you get on it. Immediately, you feel wonderful. You love the feeling of floating on the water. The raft is plush and very comfortable. First, you lie on your back and feel the water move you along, in a gentle back and forth motion. The sun is warming your body, and you feel very relaxed and very safe. You decide to slowly turn over on your stomach and look through the secret window. Below you is a world full of beautiful sea life.

Coral of all different bright colors—orange, pink, and green—lines the ocean floor. You see starfish on some of the coral. Magical fish swim by underneath you—purple, yellow, and pink fish—all different colors. Stingrays glide by and you love to see the shape of their bodies change as they swim in the water. The longer you look, the more relaxed you feel. You are not holding onto any thoughts—you are just being in the moment, and you are very calm. Focus on what you see and how you feel. Your back feels warm and soothed by the sun, and you feel a slight ocean breeze flowing over you. Take a moment to enjoy this feeling of relaxation.

In just a minute, I will count to 10, and I want you to imagine yourself climbing up a set of stairs. With each step, you become more and more alert, but still very relaxed. At the top of the stairs, there will be an archway. You will walk through the archway and then you will be back in your own room, taking with you all the feelings of relaxation.

One, take the first step.
Two, take the second step.
Three, take the third step.
Four, take the fourth step.
Five, take the fifth step.
Six, take the sixth step,
Seven, take the seventh step.
Eight, take the eighth step.
Nine, take the ninth step.
And ten, take the tenth step.

Walk through the archway and gently open your eyes. You are back in your own room. Remind yourself that you can become this relaxed anytime you'd like, and it will only take 5 minutes!

Mindfulness Meditation

Mindfulness has gained a lot of attention in the recent years, proving to help children (and adults) with stress and anxiety management. It has even begun to be integrated into the curriculum at some schools. Mindfulness is essentially the act of being aware, fully aware, of yourself, your experience, and the environment around you. It involves being fully present in the exact moment you are in right now.

Meditation is the practice of quieting the mind and entering into the perceptual field of awareness (it implies that mindfulness is also happening). When one is meditating, he is simply tuning into his body and then extending his awareness into the space around him; there are no thoughts and the focus is simply on this moment. With regular practice, deeper states of awareness can be attained; eventually, there can be a blissful state of timelessness and beyond-the-body awareness. To help with grounding oneself in the moment, one starts by observing the sounds and space around him (usually with closed eyes). Staying in this state of perception, he then expands awareness into the room, and the space begins to feel like energy around him. With extended awareness into this space, a deeper sense of consciousness is experienced. In this thoughtless state, there can be an intense calmness and stillness; this is the pure awareness of being.

Although many think of meditation as a skill to acquire and something to learn, it is actually just a return to the most natural state we can be in; it is how we were born—into a state of direct awareness, with no thought and no reflection. Children are closer to this state than adults, and usually can "learn" how to meditate with greater ease.

There are different types of meditation; the type I encourage and teach to children is mindfulness meditation. Mindfulness meditation is being fully aware and entering in the "field of awareness" without thought. Because anxiety presents as anxious thoughts (worries) and often distracts a child from the moment she is in, practicing mindfulness and mindfulness meditation provides another tool for managing anxiety. When you are in the present moment, you realize that you are OK and nothing is threatening you. The more one practices meditation, the more accessible this state of awareness will be. Knowing how to meditate and practicing regularly will end up discouraging kids from distracting themselves from the anxiety and will discourage avoidance behavior, as they will be better able to "sit with" and tolerate the discomfort that comes from facing their fears.

I recommend that you teach your child how to do mindfulness meditation. First, go through the explanation of mindfulness meditation provided in your child's book. Tell her there is no such thing as "doing it right," as it is not about "doing" anything; rather, it is relaxing into a natural state of being. Start with a 10-minute practice each day, ideally before bedtime. Gradually, your child may want to meditate for longer periods, and a 20–30 minute period is ideal.

MINDFULNESS MEDITATION SCRIPT (READ SLOWLY)

Find a comfortable space to practice; you can sit back or lie down. Close your eyes. We are going to practice mindfulness meditation (pause). When you were born, you were born into a state of awareness: There was no thinking and no reflecting—you simply just perceived and noticed what was around you. This practice is like that—like returning to that natural state of being.

I would like you to start by grounding yourself in your body. Bring all of your attention and focus to the center of your body, just below your belly button. Focus on the breath: Notice how your belly rises and falls with each incoming and outgoing breath. As you do this, if any thoughts come up, just allow them to float by you. Don't focus on them by bringing them toward you or by pushing them away, just let them float on by. Anything important will come back later. Keep the focus on your lower belly and your breath.

(Once your child seems calm and relaxed, continue with the script.)

Now I'd like you to extend your awareness into the space around you—into the room we are in. Just extend your awareness and notice any sounds, movements, and vibrations. (Point out any sounds or movements they might hear, such as "notice the sound of the clock, and the vibrations of the air conditioning.") Just notice what is around you. Feel the space around you and extend into it (long pause). Anytime thoughts come up, you can return your attention to the center of your body and the focus on your breath.

(Once your child seems to be in a calm and thoughtless state, continue with the script.)

Now I'd like you to deepen your awareness. Go a little deeper and extend beyond this room—expand your awareness to what is outside this room, this building, to the land around you. Keep extending and deepening your awareness. (Allow your child to settle into this "space" without disruption, so she can stay in it until she naturally starts talking or opens her eyes.)

(After 10 minutes or longer if there is time and she is still "in it," finish the script.)

When you are ready, you can gently open your eyes. Slowly come back into this room. Good job.

Once the practice is over, ask your child how it was for her: How did it feel? Did she have any thoughts come up? Did she notice her body when she was extending? What sounds did she notice? Keep practicing and reminding her that even if she doesn't get it immediately, it will come with continued practice. Even if you, the parent, haven't experienced anything from the exercise, keep doing the practice for your child.

Yoga

Yoga is incredibly beneficial when it comes to helping your child be in the moment and learning how to relax. When in a yoga pose, he is focused on that pose and the mind and body are one. When I'm in a handstand against the wall, I am not thinking at all; rather I am focusing on the handstand and fully in my body. Yoga comes from Sanskrit and means "to join" or "unity." I couldn't imagine a better form of relaxation for children (and adults) with anxiety, as it aims to bring oneness to the mind and body. When we are anxious, we are stuck in our minds. The more practice we have of bringing our bodies into it, the less anxious we will feel.

For young children (10 and under), I use *Yoga Pretzels,* which are a series of color cards that teach the pose by explaining the four steps to get into it. Most kids get excited about learning from the cards and there is no opposition to practicing. Older kids should watch a video or be presented with the challenge of trying some of the positions. Taking a yoga class is always ideal, and more and more studios are offering family yoga or yoga for kids.

When introducing yoga to your child, keep it light at first; but the ultimate goal is for him to use yoga as an avenue to a deep state of calmness and mind-body union, which comes with regular, consistent practice. There are many forms of yoga; I personally practice the Iyengar method, which focuses on facilitating alignment and strength.

The following are three popular poses that are simple to practice:

1. Standing Mountain Pose:
   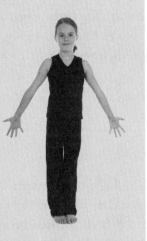
   Stand with your feet hip-width apart and your arms down by your sides. Stand up nice and tall and very straight with your shoulders back. Try to get your chest to lift up, as if someone is pulling your chest up with a string that is attached to it.

   Now turn your palms facing out, away from you. Slowly raise your arms, keeping your elbows straight if you can. Once your arms are all the way up, your hands will be facing one another, and your fingers will be reaching up toward the sky. Stretch up and reach up as high as you can, while keeping your feet planted firmly into the floor. Try to encourage your upper spine to move into your body and your shoulder blades to move closer together.

   Continue to reach up with your fingertips, and push your feet down into the floor, as if your feet were the roots of a tree (your leg muscles should become tight as you do this). Your upper body is stretching up while your lower body is pushing down. As you do this, feel confident about yourself and feel your body opening and lengthening as you stretch and stretch.

2. Downward-Facing Dog Pose:
   Lie facedown on the floor, bend your elbows, and put your hands down on the floor next to your armpits (or chest).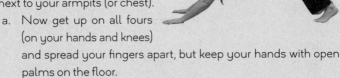
   a. Now get up on all fours (on your hands and knees) and spread your fingers apart, but keep your hands with open palms on the floor.
   b. Now lift up onto your feet, standing mainly on your toes, lifting your hips up, and keeping your hands on the floor. Your hands should be shoulder-width apart.
   c. Continue to lift your hips up and stretch your back. Continue to spread your fingers apart and push your hands against the floor to encourage more lengthening in your spine and more lift in your hips. Hips up, hips up. Feel the stretch.
   d. Very good! Now gently come back down onto all fours, lie back down on your stomach, and relax.

3. Child's Pose:
   Lie facedown on the floor, and touch your big toes together while sitting on the heels of your feet.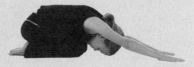
   a. Now spread your knees apart so your knees go out toward the side.
   b. Lay your chest on the floor and let your belly sink down toward the floor as well. Your thighs and knees should be out to the side.
   c. Stretch your arms and fingers out in front of you with your arms lifting up a few inches above the floor and your fingertips touching the floor. As you do this, try to get your upper back and upper spine to come into your body. Feel the stretch.
   d. Now bring your arms down by your sides, with your hands (palms facing up) resting on the floor alongside or below your feet. Just let your entire body relax and rest. Let go of any tension in your body.

Stress Management

Managing daily stress is essential in reducing overall anxiety and lowering one's baseline. In order to teach your child about stress management, she will learn about the "beaker" analogy. A beaker is used to represent someone's stress level. Everyone always has some fluid in the beaker, which signifies the daily stressors, like forgetting to turn in homework or, for adults, forgetting to pay a bill on time.

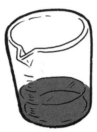

When additional events occur, such as getting a bad grade on a test, or events related to your child's anxiety disorder, the beaker level can go way up.

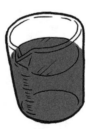

Once someone's beaker is at the top, it only takes something small, *any little thing*, to cause it to overflow. When our beakers overflow, we explode—have a meltdown, scream, yell, panic, and cry, whatever. It's up to your child to lower his own beaker level (and it is up to you, the parent, to monitor your own). Although you may help your child feel better at times, you want to encourage your child to take responsibility for his emotions—this promotes the skill of self-regulation, or learning how to manage his reaction to different events.

Here are some ideas on what your child can do to lower his beaker level:

1. Sleep well (consistent bedtime and wake time).
2. Eat well.
3. Exercise.
4. Do yoga.
5. Do relaxation.
6. Express his feelings appropriately.
7. Take a hot bath, and add bubbles if he likes.
8. Do 100 jumping jacks or push-ups (after that she'll feel too exhausted to be stressed!).
9. Write in a journal—write about what is bothering him and what he can do to make it better.
10. Paint a picture or do an art project.
11. Play an instrument.
12. Play with a pet (dog, cat).
13. Distract herself by reading a book or watching TV or a movie.
14. Call a friend.
15. Play outside.

Your child's book encourages your child to come up with additional ways that personally help him to feel better and less anxious. For all children, it is beneficial to promote a healthy diet, as there is a lot of research on the relationship between food and mood/emotional well-being (in addition to physical health). A diet free of processed foods and low in gluten and dairy (which can cause inflammation), but high in fruit, vegetables, and nuts and other low-glycemic foods will help. Processed foods and simple carbohydrates (bread, wheat pasta, mac and cheese, soda, candy, cookies, pastries, etc.) end up spiking the blood sugar and then it comes down quickly, often times creating an unbalanced mood state. Low glycemic foods take longer to break down, so one has more consistent energy without the up-and-down trend. There are a lot of great books out there on children's nutrition, but I personally have found Dr. Joel Fuhrman's *Disease-Proof Your Child: Feeding Kids Right* to be outstanding (see more recommendations in Resources under Nutrition and Dietary).

In your child's book, space is allotted for him to write down other ways that he can lower his beaker level. Because the exercise at the end of this chapter in your child's book involves a discussion on how you, his parent, manages stress, write down *your* ideas on how you can lower *your own* beaker on the lines below:

_____

_____

_____

_____

_____

_____

_____

_____

_____

Finally, it is important to create a balanced schedule/routine so that your child stays on top of schoolwork and other obligations, as this is helpful in reducing worry associated with getting everything done. I also recommend that children *and adults* have one day each week that is free from doing *any* schoolwork (or work), because everyone needs a break and one day each week that focuses on relaxing and have fun. It is essential that children have time to play and to be creative; unstructured time allows for creativity and creativity allows another opportunity for developing self-confidence. Nurturing your child's social needs also is recommended.

Chapter 3 EXERCISE

Tips for Parents

1. The exercise below includes a discussion topic for you and your child. You will need to be prepared to share ways in which you personally manage your own stress, and what you do to relax and calm down. Try to generate examples that your child can relate to, such as lying on a blanket under a tree, going to the zoo, and so forth.

2. When helping your child practice relaxation, try to create the right environment for your child to feel comfortable. For example, find a space in your home (or outside) where there is minimal or no noise, where the temperature is neutral, and where your child can really relax. Some parents have made a ritual out of it for their child: dimming the lights, lighting candles, and lying on blankets or mats on the floor. The best part is this will offer an opportunity for you to relax as well!

Practice Relaxation

Your exercise this week includes:
1. A topic question for you and your parent to talk about.
2. Making a calm breathing note card.
3. Practicing your relaxation 5 days this week.

Try not to think of practicing the relaxation as a chore, but as something that feels very good that you can look forward to doing. Knowing how to relax is one of the most important tools you will use when we get to the "facing your fears" part. Your parent will help you by practicing with you over the week.

Discussion Topic

Talk to your parents about what makes them feel relaxed—what they do to calm down and manage stress. Tell them what makes you feel relaxed and what you think can help you calm down. Your parents might want to know what they can do to help you feel less stressed.

1. Use one note card to write down how to do calm breathing. Make your note card look like this one:

> **Calm Breathing**
>
> In → nose → count of 4
> Hold → count of 4
> Out → mouth → count of 4

Then on the back, make yours look like this:

> **Calm Breathing**
>
> Breathe in and out through only one nostril. Hold your other nostril closed and close your mouth.
> Count of 10 in and count of 10 out.

2. Practice relaxation! Check off the days that you practiced and what type of relaxation you did in the chart below:

Day of the Week	Calm Breathing	Progressive Muscle Relaxation (PMR)	Relaxing Imagery	Mindfulness Meditation	Yoga
Monday					
Tuesday					
Wednesday					
Thursday					
Friday					
Saturday					
Sunday					

Try to do at least one technique a day and to try each technique at least once this week. If you choose to listen to an app or CD track, check which type of strategy was used.

EXERCISE

4

Conquer Your Worries

"What if I can't finish all of this homework? There is so much to do. I don't even know where to start. There is no way I will finish," thought Kimberly when she sat down to do her homework. She also worried about break-ins, being kidnapped, and her dog escaping. Kimberly's mom helped her make a list of her worries, and Kimberly realized that they were the same worries almost every day. She scheduled "worry time" and recorded her worries on her mom's phone and she listened back to the recording over and over until she started to worry less overall. She began to label her worries as "anxiety" and started to talk back to them. Kimberly's mom also helped her learn that the anticipatory anxiety was not a good predictor of what was to come.

> "When I look back on all these worries, I remember the story of the old man who said on his deathbed that he had a lot of trouble in his life, most of which never happened."
> —Winston Churchill

IN this chapter, you and your child will learn how to get rid of worries. Worries are thoughts (this chapter and Chapter 5 are about the "thoughts" part of anxiety), and as the quote above illustrates, most worries are a waste of time (although just knowing that is not enough to get rid of them). Worry breeds self-doubt, which can cause a negative impact on your child's self-esteem, especially if the worrying is chronic and limits what they can do. This chapter will help your child learn how to deal with his worries and ultimately to feel more confident. A primary goal of this program is to promote a sense of empowerment in your child; this will be accomplished largely by having your child face his fears, but also by learning to not be organized by worrying thoughts.

There are several strategies to conquer worry (each of these are covered in your child's book):

- ▶ understanding the two types of worry,
- ▶ asking yourself two things,
- ▶ positive self-talk,
- ▶ talking back to the anxiety,
- ▶ challenging anticipatory anxiety
- ▶ schedule "worry time,"
- ▶ worry tapes, and
- ▶ uncertainty training.

Understanding the Two Types of Worry: Useful and Useless Worry

One way to challenge worries is to differentiate between those that are useful or helpful and those that are useless. As you probably know, some amount of anxiety is often beneficial, as it motivates you to get things done in a timely manner. **Useful** worry, therefore, helps you be more productive without causing a negative physiological reaction (e.g., rapid heart rate, tight muscles, upset stomach, or avoidance behavior). **Useless** worry is worry that causes an interruption, or impairment, in your ability to get things done. In fact, this type of worry often can prevent you from being productive and often results in a negative physiological reaction (e.g., rapid heart rate, tight muscles, upset stomach).

In your child's book, she will learn to label useless worry as "just the anxiety talking," (and the exercise at the end of this chapter is designed to help her with this process) and something to get rid of. Later on, through facing her fears, your child will learn that there was nothing to worry about in the first place, confirming that her worry was useless. She also will learn that worrying makes her feel a false sense of control. It does this by making her feel like she is doing something to deal with her anxiety (i.e., worrying). In fact, just the opposite is true—worrying actually strengthens her anxiety about the situation and makes the event seem worse. In addition, she worries and then nothing bad happens, so the worry is associated with a positive outcome; this strengthens the worry process and increases the likelihood that she'll worry in the future.

Asking Yourself Two Things

When you are worried, ask yourself the following two questions:
1. What is the worst thing that could happen?
2. Could I handle it?

The answer is *always* "yes." Remind your child that he can handle anything that comes his way, and that you can handle anything that comes your way. Reinforce that although bad things can happen, there is nothing in life that he cannot handle. This supports a resilient mindset—the notion that we can manage obstacles and overcome them, not be defined by them.

Positive Self-Talk

Self-talk is what you say to yourself. Children who are anxious often engage in negative self-talk. Some examples include:
"I can't do it."
"I can't handle this."
"I won't be OK."
"It's going to be terrible!"
"I need to be with my mom or dad to feel safe."

"This is too scary."

"I'm too nervous to do this."

These kinds of statements strengthen your child's fears and anxiety. However, if those thoughts are replaced with or challenged by positive self-talk, particularly when your child is being exposed to an anxiety-provoking situation, he will improve his ability to cope and feel more confident about being capable of tolerating the situation. Learning how to tolerate the anxiety-provoking situation is necessary in order for habituation to occur (as mentioned in Chapter 1, habituation is the process of getting used to, or "numbing out" to something; for example, the longer you stay in a freezing cold swimming pool, the warmer the water begins to feel because you have habituated to the temperature) and positive self-talk can help.

Here are some examples of positive self-talk:

"I must face my fears to overcome them. I can do it!"

"I can handle this. I am nervous, but I am OK."

"I am scared, but I am safe."

"I am OK. Everything will work out."

"I can handle whatever comes my way."

"I can change the way I think to change the way I feel."

"It is my choice to be calm or be nervous. I am choosing to be calm. Let me start by calming my breath."

"Anxiety is not an accurate predictor of what's to come. Anxiety is just an unpleasant feeling."

"It is just the anxiety talking; I don't have to listen to it."

"What would someone without anxiety think in this situation? What would they do?"

"What would someone without OCD think in this situation? What would they do?"

"What would someone who is completely confident do in this situation?"

Here are some additional examples of older children/teens:

"I cannot allow anxiety to make decisions for me."

"I cannot allow anxiety to influence my behavior or the behavior of my family."

"It's me versus the anxiety. Each time I listen to the anxiety and let it rule my life, it gets stronger. Each time I make decisions based on my values and not the anxiety, I get stronger."

"Courage comes after slaying the dragon. Once I face my fears, I will realize I can do it."

"I've never regretted facing my fears."

"I have to 'sit with' and tolerate the discomfort."

"I will manage my stress by taking one step at a time and only focusing on the task in front of me."

"I can take breaks to relax and calm my body. Managing stress is part of being a healthy, successful student."

We want to encourage kids to use positive self-talk, even though they likely won't initially believe what they are telling themselves. With practice, your child will see that these statements are true! The goal is for him to find 2–3 favorites from this list and memorize them so they are readily accessible to use when faced with an anxiety-provoking situation. The more he uses positive self-talk, the more he will feel like he can handle situations that make him feel anxious.

Talking Back to the Anxiety

Part of self-talk is learning how to "talk back" to the anxiety. By doing this, your child externalizes the anxiety. Externalizing the anxiety allows your child to see the anxiety as something separate from her. This process of externalization enables your child to (1) identify her anxious thoughts and feelings more accurately,

(2) challenge these thoughts and feelings and adopt a more balanced way of thinking about anxiety-provoking situations, and (3) face her fears. It is important that your child realize that she and the anxiety are not the same; that the anxiety is a separate thing, even though it often feels like it is part of her. This is challenging because one of the symptoms of anxiety is anxious thoughts; yet anxious children have many other nonanxious thoughts that are mixed in. Because anxious thoughts are mixed in with general (nonanxious) thoughts, it makes it harder to distinguish the anxious thoughts as just "symptoms," since they are often experienced as regular thoughts. The next chapter will address this further.

In your child's book, she is told to think of the anxiety as external (outside of her), as something separate. When she has a scary thought, she should say to herself, "It is just the anxiety talking" and remind herself that she doesn't need to listen to it. For most children, this alone won't get rid of the thoughts; they also will need to desensitize to the thoughts by playing the worry recording (see below), but it will help in challenging them. Emphasize that the alternative is that if she listens to these worries, the anxiety will become stronger and it will win. But, if she doesn't listen to it, *she* will become stronger and *she* will win.

Challenging Anticipatory Anxiety

Anticipatory anxiety is when you feel nervous or worried about something before it actually happens. For example, you tell your child that you will be going out of town for the weekend, and she becomes extremely upset and worried at that moment when you tell her. Maybe she will ask you numerous questions about your plans, or maybe she'll begin to cry and protest your trip. This is called *anticipatory anxiety*, because she is anticipating (or waiting for) something to happen that she perceives as scary. Most anxiety is, in fact, just anticipatory anxiety. Most children end up realizing that their perceived catastrophe was not that bad after all, or that it was difficult at first but then became more comfortable for them (due to habituation). Worrying is about what they fear is *going* to happen, not something that already has happened!

As explained in your child's book, here are the three steps he should learn in order to deal or cope with anticipatory anxiety:

1. Label your worries and scary feelings as "anticipatory anxiety." Say to yourself, "It is just anticipatory anxiety, and anxiety is not a good predictor of what's to come."

2. Replace these thoughts with healthier, more balanced thoughts. Use positive self-talk to reassure yourself that you will be OK and that you can handle what comes your way (e.g., "I will be OK and I can handle what comes my way").

3. Remind yourself to "be proactive." Proactive people do not allow anxiety to make decisions for them or influence their behavior (although reactive people do).

Schedule "Worry Time"

Another technique used to conquer worrying is to schedule *worry time* for your child. Worry time consists of setting aside a set amount of time, ranging from 10–20 minutes, in which your child intentionally worries. This time is planned out in advance and can be scheduled once or twice a day, depending on how often your child worries (more frequent worrying should involve two worry time sessions). The purpose of this is threefold: First, it helps to encourage your child to externalize her worries by "getting them out," but in a structured way versus randomly; second, it helps to encourage your child to delay worrying until the scheduled time and therefore gives her practice with compartmentalizing her worries; and third, she will begin to see the repetitiveness and uselessness of her worries, as they typically will be the same themes from day to day.

When helping your child structure the worry time, the goal is for her to use the whole time and not stop short. Even if she runs out of things to worry about, she should keep trying to think of things to worry about and if nothing comes up, she should just stay there until the time runs out. This helps create the frame for the worry time and highlights the uselessness of worrying.

There are a few different ways to "worry" during worry time. Your child can choose to simply verbalize her worries out loud to a parent, or she can write them down or type them up in a list format. Another option is to make a worry tape, which is actually the best technique to use for conquering worries and repetitive anxious thoughts (see next section).

Worry Tapes

In the world of business, you are supposed to underpromise and overdeliver, but when it comes to the effectiveness of worry tapes, I will do the opposite of the underpromise part and assure you that I have had 100% success with worry tapes (also called *loop tapes*). Every child (and adult) that I have treated has desensitized to the worries on their worry recordings. It is a simple principle: With the repetition of hearing yourself say the worries that naturally come up in your head over and over, they eventually lose their power. The thoughts become boring, unalarming, and nontriggering.

When making a worry tape, you can use a digital recorder (or an easier option if you have a smartphone is to use the voice recorder option; for iPhones, use the Voice Memos). Many children benefit from first typing out a script to read from: They can list their worries and then read from the list while recording them. Some children will do well with "free associating" and just verbalizing their worries naturally (without a script) and recording them this way. It is very important for your child to record the worries how they actually sound in her head (e.g., instead of recording "Sometimes I worry that a dog will bite me," she would record "What if that dog bites me?")

Once the recording is at least 1 minute long, your child can begin to listen to it. As she starts to listen, her anxiety will go up at first, before it gets better. She should just "sit with" and tolerate the discomfort, which is very important, as the goal is also to desensitize to the negative feelings (usually anxiety) elicited by the thoughts. She may also have additional worries come up; when this happens, she can add these worries to the recording and make a longer loop. Most children will have 2–3 different recordings that they use during the practice period. The only caveat to this is if your child has OCD with the ritual of the need to confess, it can become a neutralizing ritual/compulsion to keep adding to the recording; in this case, additional recordings should not be made more than 4–5 times.

The goal is for your child to listen to the worry tape for at least 10 minutes a day for 2–4 weeks (e.g., if it is a 2-minute long recording, she would listen 5 times in a row). For more severe anxiety, it should be 20 minutes a day and may require 6 weeks of practice. She must stay focused and pay attention when listening, as this is necessary for desensitization to occur. For children with ADHD or who just have a hard time keeping their focus on listening to the recording, you can break it down into two 5-minute practices per day. Anytime they find their attention starting to drift, they should pause the tape and perhaps stand up and stretch then resume listening with better focus.

The goal is for your child to habituate to the thoughts, not to be OK with the content of the thoughts. For example, let's say your child has separation anxiety and constantly worries about something bad happening to Mom. Her worry tape will include thoughts such as "What if something bad happens to Mom? What is she gets in a car accident and dies?" The goal is not to be OK with this horrific outcome (the content of the thoughts), rather, the goal is to become desensitized to just the thought itself so that it doesn't end up triggering the anxious feeling. When this happens, the content of the thought—the situation she is worrying about and imagining—will not be thought about at all (it will not even be considered); the thought itself will not solicit any negative feelings or reactions.

You will know when your child has habituated to the thoughts on the worry tape when he (1) has no reaction to listening or no anxiety listening and (2) when he complains that listening is so boring! When your child complains of boredom when listening to his anxious thoughts, we have reached success.

The great part about worry tapes is how easy and effective they are to use. They become a strategy that can be utilized in the future if new worries arise. I have had follow-up appointments with many kids who told me that they made more worry tapes for new worries that popped up and it worked, and they didn't need to return to therapy to be successful in treating their worries!

Finally, there is a contradiction between worry tapes and self-talk, which I would like to clarify. Worry tapes and uncertainty training recordings (next section) are used as a planned strategy to change your child's experience of her anxious thoughts; worry time, worry tapes, and uncertainty training are all practiced at a planned time, with the purpose of reframing the anxious thoughts. The goal is for children to habituate to the scary thoughts, not to tell themselves that they will be OK (rather, to desensitize to the thoughts about bad things happening). Self-talk, on the other hand, offers your child a tool to be able to cope when in an anxiety-provoking situation. When we get to the behavioral component and challenge the anxiety-provoking situations by gradually facing them, your child will use self-talk to help herself cope with the practice exposures. When facing her fears, she will use positive self-talk to get through it.

Uncertainty Training

Anxiety and worries are generally about what *might* happen, as opposed to what actually will happen. For this reason, children who learn how to tolerate uncertainty—to be OK with not knowing what will happen, or not knowing for sure—are better able to conquer their worries. Uncertainty training teaches children how to tolerate uncertainty. The same principle that underlies the effectiveness of worry tapes applies to uncertainty training: with repeated practice, the thoughts end up become boring and unalarming. Again, the goal is to desensitize to the anxious thoughts about what could, or might, happen. Dr. Robert Leahy described this technique in his 2006 book *The Worry Cure*.

When practicing tolerating uncertainty, the child makes a second loop recording, but this time instead of just listing the worries and the "what-if" thoughts, he repeats: "It is always possible that something bad will happen to Mom. It's possible that she will get in a car accident and it's always possible that she will die." I tend to have children do a regular worry tape and then use the same thoughts to make an uncertainty training tape. This way, the child listens to both (one after the other), which is incredibly effective at having them overcome and master their worries. They can listen as part of the 10–20 minute daily practice. Although no one likes to do these recordings (including parents), they are completely effective at changing the thoughts and taking away their power over your child. In fact, the worry tapes and uncertainty training recordings are often necessary to get the child to get rid of his anxious ruminations.

Chapter 4 EXERCISE

Tips for Parents

1. When helping your child make the self-talk note cards, try to make them as specific to her fears as possible. The more personalized they are, the more effective they will be in helping your child manage her specific fears.

2. Self-talk statements are designed to help your child be able to effectively cope with the anxiety-provoking situation. In addition, self-talk often challenges his anxious automatic thoughts. Table 2 presents a list of sample self-talk statements organized by type of anxiety disorder, which you can use as a guide for helping your child make his note cards.

3. While assisting your child in making her worry tape, encourage her to express all the scary thoughts that she is likely going to be reluctant to share. Empathize with how hard it is to verbalize the scary thoughts, but assure her that if an anxious thought is in her head, it's worth putting in on the recording. Just saying it doesn't mean anything— she's already thinking it! Even though making and listening to the recording is hard at first, it is the key to getting rid of the anxious thoughts. Assure her of the effectiveness of the technique and praise her for being brave for making it. Again, it is useful to first write out all of the worries that will go on the recording, and then read from the list to make the loop tape. As the parent, you can model it by making the recording first, but the actual one that she will use to desensitize to should be in her voice. The thoughts should be recorded by her, in the way that the thoughts sound in her head (so it should sound like "what if we have a break in and someone hurts us?" rather than "sometimes I worry that someone will break in"). Also, you can use the

EXERCISE

Table 2
Self-Talk Note Cards Guide

Type of Anxiety Disorder	Positive Self-Talk Statement
Generalized Anxiety Disorder	"I can control my body. I can slow my breathing and calm my body." "It's just the anxiety talking. Thoughts have no power unless I give them power." "I can handle whatever comes my way." "Uncertainty is a part of life. I need to 'sit with' and tolerate the anxiety."
Separation Anxiety Disorder	"I have to be OK on my own. It will feel scary at first, but then it will get better." "I am scared, but I am safe." "I know it's hard to separate from _____ (mom, dad), but I know I can do it. I know just how to soothe myself. I can _____ (do relaxation, bake with my babysitter, color, take a bath)." "Whether Mom/Dad is here or not, I'm safe at home."
Social Anxiety Disorder	"How would someone who isn't anxious think or act in this situation?" "It is OK to look nervous in front of others. Everyone feels nervous from time to time." "Once I'm there, I'll be fine. I can go for just part of it as a start." "What would someone who is totally confident in this situation think? What would they do?"
Specific Phobia	"(Dogs are, flying is, blood draws are) not dangerous. So many people wouldn't (have them as pets, travel, give blood) if they were. My fears are irrational." "I have to face my fears and touch this dog. Behavior changes happen first and thoughts change second." "I must face my fears of dogs/flying/blood; I must do this to win and overcome my fears. I know I can do this."

EXERCISE

Type of Anxiety Disorder	Positive Self-Talk Statement
Obsessive-Compulsive Disorder	"It is just the OCD talking; if I listen and do what it says, it will win and I will lose. If I don't listen, I will win and the OCD will lose." "It's only a thought, just a thought. Thoughts have no power unless I give them power. Thoughts are symptoms of OCD." "Each time I _____ (check, touch, count, etc), the OCD becomes stronger and wins." "OCD creates self-doubt. I have to resist the urge to check, count, ask, tell, etc."
Panic Disorder	"I don't need to be afraid of a panic attack. It feels uncomfortable, but it is not dangerous." "I can handle feeling anxious." "Panic attacks are hard to handle, but I can do it. The panic will get better soon; no one gets stuck in a panic attack." "Nothing bad is happening to me. It just feels scary." "I can leave the situation for a few minutes, until I calm down, but then I must go back to the situation. I'm not going to let the panic interfere with what I am doing." "Panic is a fear of fear and nothing else. I have to face my fear of fear!" "The panic is in *me*, not the situation. There is nothing magical about leaving the situation."

thoughts that she lists in the "When my anxiety talks, it says . . ." exercise for the recording.

4. Try to get your child to practice relaxation at least three times this week (on three different days over the week) and ensure that several types of relaxation are practiced. At least one of the three times should be on his own, without you present, as he ultimately needs to be able to use these skills

on his own (e.g., when he is facing his fears). Encourage your child to use the calm breathing exercises anytime he feels or seems anxious or tense. If you have trouble getting your child to practice the relaxation or to do any of the exercises in this book, refer to Chapter 9, which discusses how to motivate your child to participate in the program.

Self-Talk Note Cards and Worry Tapes

Your exercise this week includes:
1. Making 8–10 self-talk note cards.
2. Making a list: "When the anxiety talks, it says . . . "
3. Making a recording (either worry tape or uncertainty training or both).
4. Keep practicing your relaxation (try to do it at least three times this week).

Self-Talk Note Cards

When making your note cards, you can use different colored index cards and you can add stickers to the note cards if you'd like. You can write them or have your parent write them—it's your choice. You will make seven note cards like the ones below, and also make three of your own (you can make more if you'd like, but try to make at least three extra cards). The ones that you make on your own should be specific to you; they should be things that you can say to yourself that will help with your own specific worries and anxieties. Your mom or dad will help you with what to write.

EXERCISE

Here are seven note cards to make (make yours look just like these, with your own self-talk included):

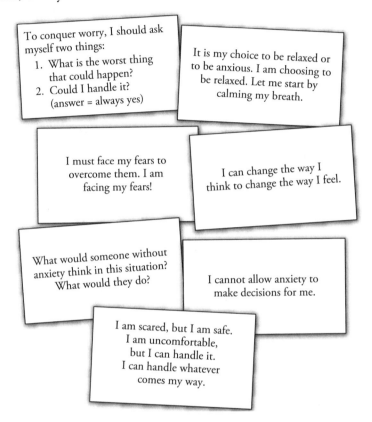

To conquer worry, I should ask myself two things:
1. What is the worst thing that could happen?
2. Could I handle it? (answer = always yes)

It is my choice to be relaxed or to be anxious. I am choosing to be relaxed. Let me start by calming my breath.

I must face my fears to overcome them. I am facing my fears!

I can change the way I think to change the way I feel.

What would someone without anxiety think in this situation? What would they do?

I cannot allow anxiety to make decisions for me.

I am scared, but I am safe. I am uncomfortable, but I can handle it. I can handle whatever comes my way.

It's the Anxiety Talking

Remember James, the boy who was afraid of snakes? Well, when his anxiety was talking, it said things like:

"Snakes are scary and they bite."

"Don't go near the bushes, because a snake could be in there."

"That rustling sound was a snake."

"You can't go near snakes—they are the worst!"

James had to learn how to talk back to his anxiety, and he did this by knowing when his anxiety was talking to him and choosing not to listen to it! He told himself that the anxiety was wrong;

then he told himself different things to help himself be able to face his fears. For example, he told himself that the rustling sound was most likely a squirrel or a bird. He reminded himself that most snakes don't bite humans. This is how he was able to face his fears and overcome his fear of snakes.

In the space below, write in some of the things that the anxiety says when you are feeling scared or anxious:

"When my anxiety talks, it says . . ."

_____

_____

_____

_____

_____

_____

_____

_____

_____

Make a Recording

Write down all of your worries, just as they sound in your head. You can use what you wrote above for "When my anxiety talks, it says . . ." Then record your worries on a phone or digital recorder (have your parent help you with the set up). When doing the recording, remember to make it sound exactly as it sounds in your head. For example, let's say you are afraid of a dog jumping on you, you would record the thought as it sounds when you think it: "What if that dog jumps on me?" (you wouldn't say "Sometimes I worry that a dog will jump on me"). We want it to sound just like it sounds in your head, so the recording should be in your voice.

EXERCISE

EXERCISE

You can do a worry loop tape or an uncertainty training recording ("It is always possible that a dog will jump on me"), or both. It is best to do both and then listen to both recordings. Remember that it gets worse before it gets easier and that while many people don't like to hear the worries on a recording, when you listen to it over and over for 10–20 minutes a day for 2–4 weeks, your worries will become boring to you. Doing this works 100% of the time!

_____

_____

_____

_____

_____

_____

_____

_____

Practice Relaxation

Use the chart in the previous chapter to check off the days that you practiced and what type of relaxation you did.

5

Changing Your Thoughts

In working toward overcoming her anxiety, Kimberly was taught that she had to change the way she thinks to change the way she feels. So, if she was to start feeling less anxious, she would need to start thinking differently. Kimberly did a lot of "What if . . ." thinking, which she learned was called **catastrophizing**, a thinking mistake. She also made things seem worse, or a bigger deal, than they were, a thinking mistake called **magnifying**, and had to do things her way or refused to do them at all, which was called **all-or-nothing** thinking. Kimberly began to catch herself making these thinking mistakes and challenged herself by trying to think differently and in a more flexible manner. Her parents helped her identify when she was making a thinking mistake, as they gently pointed it out to her when it happened.

I N this chapter, you and your child will learn about the different types of cognitive distortions or "thinking errors." You also will learn how to help your child change his anxious thoughts and beliefs and change his relationship with his thoughts by learning detached mindfulness (as a reminder, this chapter also is about the thoughts part of anxiety).

Let's start by understanding the connection between your thoughts and feelings. The way your child thinks about a situation impacts the way he will feel about it and how he behaves in response. For example, if he thinks that playing with your neighbor's dog is enjoyable and fun, he will feel excited and play with the dog. Yet, if he thinks that playing with your neighbor's dog is scary and frightening, he will feel anxious and scared and avoid playing with the dog.

The following examples are directly from your child's book:

Situation →	Thoughts →	Feelings →	Actions
You are in front of your house and your neighbor is outside with her dog.	I really like dogs and can't wait to play with Charlie. He's so cute!	Excited Happy Eager	Go outside and pet Charlie.

Situation →	Thoughts →	Feelings →	Actions
You are in front of your house and your neighbor is outside with her dog.	Dogs are so scary! I hope he doesn't come near me. If he comes toward me, I'll run inside!	Anxious Nervous Scared	Stay inside or run away from Charlie if he comes near you.

Situation →	Thoughts →	Feelings →	Actions
You are called on in class by the teacher to answer a question.	I feel comfortable being called on. I like to share my thoughts. Maybe the teacher will like my answer.	Relaxed Calm Enthusiastic	Comfortably and naturally share your ideas.

Situation →	Thoughts →	Feelings →	Actions
You are called on in class by the teacher to answer a question.	I can't stand talking in front of the class. What if I say the wrong answer and everyone laughs and thinks I'm dumb?	Anxious Nervous Scared	Quietly say, "I don't know," or limit what you say.

Situation →	Thoughts →	Feelings →	Actions
You have a big science test tomorrow and you have been studying for 3 days.	I am prepared and will probably do well because I have been studying a lot.	Calm Self-Assured Organized	Take the test, focusing on trying your best.

Situation →	Thoughts →	Feelings →	Actions
You have a big science test tomorrow and you have been studying for 3 days.	What if I fail? What if I forget everything I know? I will be in big trouble if I fail. The test is going to be impossible!	Anxious Nervous Scared	Have trouble sleeping the night before and ask your parents for reassurance.

These examples illustrate that if something makes your child feel anxious, it has to do with the way he is thinking about it. Additionally, this means that your child can *change the way he thinks to change the way he feels*! This is an essential component to overcoming worry and anxiety. Remind him that he can do this, and that with practice, he will become proficient at it. When reviewing these concepts with your child, encourage him to consider that if the child in the above example were to change his thoughts and think like a nonanxious person, he would feel calm and relaxed and take better actions. For instance, instead of thinking about failing the science exam and getting in big trouble, he could replace these thoughts with healthier ones like "I am prepared and I will probably do well because I have been studying a lot." Initially, your child may not believe these thoughts—they will feel unfamiliar and foreign; however, with practice and time, balanced, healthy thinking will become natural and automatic.

An important part of changing thoughts is to identify the specific cognitive errors that your child is making. This also will help your child identify patterns of her thinking. Thinking mistakes consistently result in negative feelings, such as anxiety and insecurity. It is also important for your child to know that the thoughts don't have any power (the thoughts only have power if they are given power by your child or by you).

Types of Cognitive Distortions (Thinking Mistakes and Thinking Errors)

Everyone, including all children and adults, makes thinking mistakes or thinking errors. Thinking errors occur automatically and often exist outside of your child's awareness. Your child will learn that thinking errors are erroneous because they are inaccurate or irrational. In fact, most thinking errors made by your child are rooted in anxiety (and serve to reinforce anxiety). Tell your child that she should not feel bad about making thinking errors, and remind her that all children and adults make them. The following is a personal example that I share with your child in her book:

Years ago, I was visiting an island called Barbados and heard that there were really cool sea turtles in the ocean. The only thing was that you needed to take a speedboat to get to see them. Well, when the motorboat came up to the ocean shore to pick us up, I suddenly felt a rush of anxiety and fear and worry come over me. My heart started pounding, my stomach and knees felt weak, and I couldn't stop thinking about how scary it would feel going so fast on this boat—speeding along on the ocean. And I kept thinking that the boat was going so far from shore and what if it broke down and we got stuck out there? I really felt too afraid to go. I told my husband Brian that I was so nervous that I wasn't sure I could go, and told him that I might not go and he replied, "Well, you need to face your fears, just like the kids you work with," then he jumped onto the boat! I decided to take his (really my) advice and got on the boat too. The next thing I know, we are speeding along on the ocean going very fast and the funny thing was, I had no anxiety at all! Not even the tiniest amount of fear. I probably couldn't have felt afraid if I tried. I was totally calm and relaxed and loved every minute of the boat ride. I loved the feeling of the ocean air against my face, the feeling of being on a boat, traveling on water, and looking at the beautiful island as we rode by. More than all of this, swimming with the sea turtles was one of the greatest times of my life! The sea turtles were huge and so interesting to watch as they swam in their ocean. It was a magical time and it would never have happened if I didn't face my fears.

It is clear that the thoughts I had about going on the boat and my physiological reaction of anxiety were not accurate predictors of my experience on the motorboat. My thoughts were actually thinking errors and the two specific ones I made were "probability overestimations" and "catastrophizing." This is a good example of how one thought can actually represent more than one thinking error.

Below is a list of 10 different thinking errors and examples of each (these also are listed in Appendix B: Thinking Errors Quick Reference). Note that most children with anxiety disorders tend to make several thinking errors on a consistent basis. When learning about the different types, try to consider which ones you have personally made and which ones you observe your child making:

1. **Catastrophizing:** Your child expects, even visualizes disaster. She notices or hears about a potential problem and thinks, "What if . . ." the worst thing happens. She also feels like she couldn't handle it if something bad did happen.

    a.   *Example:* Your child thinks, "What if I am scared on the motorboat and won't be able to calm down? What if we get stuck out in the middle of the ocean?"

    b.   *Example:* You are going out for dinner and your child asks, "Mommy, what if something bad happens to you?"

2.   **All-or-Nothing:** Also known as black-and-white thinking, dichotomous thinking, and polarized thinking; when your child thinks in extremes and has only two categories (e.g., perfect or failure). There is no middle ground—it's either one extreme or another; thinking in an inflexible way.

    a.   *Example:* Your child feels that if he doesn't get an A on the test, then he will fail the whole class and his report card will be ruined.

    b.   *Example:* You planned on having pizza for dinner, but the pizza place closed so you brought home Chinese food instead. Your daughter is extremely upset about this and announces, "The whole day is ruined now! I didn't want Chinese!"

3.   **Filtering:** When your child focuses on the negative parts of a situation while ignoring the positive parts; she catches all of the bad parts and forgets about the good parts; she disqualifies the positive.

    a.   *Example:* Your daughter goes to a birthday party and has a great time until the end when another kid says something mean to her. When you pick her up and ask how the party was, she tells you, "It was terrible. I had the worst time!"

    b.   *Example:* Her report card arrives and she made all A's and B's but got one C in history. She is so upset and only focuses on her history grade; she ignores all of the other good grades that she earned and begins to cry about the C.

4. **Magnifying:** When your child makes something seem bigger and worse than it really is; he turns up the volume on anything bad, making it worse.

   a. *Example:* You remind your son that he has a check-up at the doctor's tomorrow after school, and he begins to cry and tells you this is the worst news he has ever heard and he hates his life!

   b. *Example:* A bug lands on your son's shirt and he screams at the top of his lungs and runs around trying to get it off.

5. **Shoulds:** Rules that your child has about the way things should be; when she uses the words *should, must,* and *ought* to show how things should be.

   a. *Example:* Your daughter forgets to hand in a homework assignment. When she hands it in the next day, her teacher marks it down to a B because it is late. She becomes very upset with herself and thinks, "I shouldn't make mistakes like this. That was so stupid of me."

   b. *Example:* Your child has her friend Mary come over to play with her and she thinks that Mary should be willing to play whatever games she picks, because they are playing at her house. Your daughter picks out Monopoly, but Mary doesn't want to play Monopoly and would rather play Clue, so your daughter becomes very upset with Mary because she believes that Mary should follow her rules. She then refuses to play anything other than Monopoly.

6. **Mind Reading:** When your child thinks she knows what others are thinking, particularly what they are thinking about her; usually she thinks that others are thinking negatively about her.

a. *Example:* When she answers a question in class, your child thinks that other kids are thinking that she is stupid and doesn't know what she is talking about.

b. *Example:* When her softball coach gives her a pointer, she believes that he thinks that she is the worst player on the team.

7. **Overgeneralization:** Your child takes a single incident and thinks that it always will be this way; something happens once and he thinks it will always happen in the same way.

a. *Example:* He gets very nervous when giving a presentation on a book report. Afterward, he comments that he is not good at giving presentations and expects that he will always feels anxious when giving them.

b. *Example:* You and your son go to an awards ceremony at his school, but he doesn't get any awards. When leaving, he tells you that he is never going to an awards ceremony again because he won't get an award anyway, so what's the point?

8. **Personalization:** When your child takes something personally, she makes it about her when it has nothing to do with her. She takes responsibility when a negative outcome occurs, without considering other factors that may have contributed to it.

a. *Example:* Your daughter walks by two girls in the lunchroom who are whispering and she thinks that they are whispering about her.

b. *Example:* She didn't receive an invitation to her friend's birthday party so she thinks that her friend must be mad at her and doesn't want to be her friend anymore.

9. **Selective Attention:** Your child pays attention to things that confirm his beliefs about something; he ignores evidence that goes against what he believes about a particular situation.
   a. *Example:* He thinks that other kids don't like him and then he tells you about the time he was teased at recess and the time when his neighbor told him that she didn't want to play with him anymore. He doesn't think about the kids who do like him or about all of the fun times he had with his friends from the soccer team.
   b. *Example:* His brother gets a new computer and he begins to think that you and his other parent don't get him anything, and how his computer is 2 years old. He doesn't think about how he recently got a new bed and that when he got his computer 2 years ago, his brother did not get one.

10. **Probability Overestimation:** Your child overestimates the likelihood that something bad will happen.
    a. *Example:* Your daughter thinks that her presentation is going to be terrible and that she will be panicked the whole time.
    b. *Example:* Your child is about to get on a motorboat and begins to think that she will be scared and anxious during the whole ride (does this sound familiar?).

It is common for certain anxiety disorders to be associated with certain thinking errors; however, any child can make any of the above thinking errors, regardless of his or her diagnosis. Table 3 specifies common thinking errors for each type of anxiety disorder.

In addition to the 10 cognitive distortions described above, there are several others that are specific to obsessive-compulsive disorder (OCD), and these are covered in the special section on OCD in Chapter 10.

Table 3
Common Thinking Errors

Type of Anxiety Disorder	Common Thinking Errors
Generalized Anxiety Disorder	Catastrophizing, All-or-Nothing, Magnifying, Filtering, Selective Attention
Separation Anxiety Disorder	Catastrophizing, Magnifying, Probability Overestimation
Social Phobia	Mind Reading, Personalization, Probability Overestimation, Shoulds, Selective Attention
Specific Phobia	Catastrophizing, Magnifying, Filtering, Probability Overestimation, Selective Attention
Obsessive-Compulsive Disorder	All-or-Nothing, Catastrophizing, Shoulds, Probability Overestimation
Panic Disorder	Catastrophizing, Probability Overestimation

Replacing Your Anxious Thoughts

After your child has identified her anxious thoughts, the next step is to change them. She can do this by replacing her thinking errors with more balanced, neutral thoughts. For example, instead of thinking that others are thinking bad things about her, she can think that most likely this is not the case. Instead of thinking about something bad happening to her mom or dad, she can think about how her parents go out to dinner all the time and are always safe; she also can remind herself that going out to dinner is a safe activity (and challenging thinking errors should be done in addition to conquer worry techniques like worry tapes). Instead of thinking that the whole day is ruined because her mom brought home Chinese food and not pizza, she can learn to think about the day more realistically and balance her disappointment about not having pizza with thoughts about how the rest of the day can be great.

To replace her thoughts, your child must "consider the facts" and ask herself, "What proof do I have that this thought is correct?" For example, what proof does she have that her mind reading is correct? How does she know that the other kids think she is stupid when she answers a question in class? How does she know how she will feel once she is speeding along the water on a motorboat? What proof does she have that her presentation will be a disaster? Even if she has given a not-so-fantastic presentation in the past, how does she know that this particular presentation will not go well? The *fact* is that she doesn't have any proof about what will happen in the future because it hasn't happened yet! Remind her that her worries are part of anticipatory anxiety; they are about future events that haven't occurred yet. The self-talk of "What would someone without anxiety think?" is also an excellent way to shift him out of his anxious thinking pattern/thinking errors.

Changing Your Relationship With Your Anxious Thoughts

An important goal when treating your child's anxiety is to get him to change his relationship with his thoughts. Thoughts don't have any power on their own—they are just thoughts. They only have power if we give them power, which means we can also take their power over us away. Detached mindfulness is a technique that is part of "metacognitive therapy," developed by Dr. Adrian Wells (2011). Metacognitive therapy, or MCT, is a type of cognitive therapy that focuses on one's relationship to his thoughts, and how he thinks (versus *what* he thinks).

The detached mindfulness technique teaches your child how to become aware (or mindful) of and separate (or detached) from his thoughts by becoming an observer of them. When you become an observer of your thoughts, you see yourself having the thoughts (the anxious thoughts) and are better able to view them as "just thoughts." You go from being a participant in your thoughts to an observer of them, which allows you to then reclassify the thoughts as just symptoms of anxiety. This allows your child to identify his worries as "just thoughts" which are "just symptoms." Whether a thought is true or not, it's just a thought and nothing else. In detached mindfulness, you don't try to change the thought itself; rather, you try to change how you experience the thought. So, we want your child to experience the thought as a symptom of, or manifestation of, anxiety, and not a real thought or real indication of anything other than anxiety. The goal is for your child to no longer examine the content of the anxious thoughts and instead be able to just see the thoughts without reacting to them.

The method I use to teach detached mindfulness is as follows: I take 10 sheets or paper and write down 10 different thoughts (seven neutral, two anxiety-provoking, and one untrue), then I have the child read the 10 thoughts three times in a row, quickly. The thoughts are arranged in a specific order, so they are mixed up (note the order below in the example). Once they read the thoughts three times in a row, they say aloud: "I can see these are just thoughts. Whether they are true or not, neutral or scary, they are just thoughts. Thoughts do not have any power unless I give them power." I will have the child practice this 1–2 times a day for 2–3 weeks depending on the severity of their anxiety.

Here are is an example of the 10 thoughts:

"I love pepperoni pizza from Ledo's. Maybe I'll have it this weekend." (N)
"The fall is my favorite season—the leaves are so amazing." (N)
"I have a big test next week and will have to study a lot for it." (N)
"What if someone breaks in and kills us all?" (A)

"Over winter break we are going to Florida—I can't wait." (N)
"I will probably join the animal rights club that's starting soon." (N)
"I'm wearing neon green socks." (U)
"My favorite books are the Harry Potter series" (N)
"What if there is another terrorist attack?" (A)
"I love my brother. We have the best time playing together." (N)

(N = neutral, A = anxiety-provoking, U = untrue)

The most brilliant feedback I received from a 13-year-old with OCD who mastered this technique was when he told me, "I think I got it. Now, when the terrible thoughts come up, I see them as if they are being typed out on a screen in front of me; I cannot really read them or know them, but I see it as just the OCD and it doesn't bother me anymore." With practice, your child can also learn to become an observer of his anxious thoughts and therefore not be affected by them.

EXERCISE

Chapter 5 EXERCISE

Tips for Parents

1. When helping your child complete this exercise, try to pick one of the less anxiety-provoking situations and one of the most anxiety-provoking situations on his ladder. If your child wants to use two of the harder situations, that is acceptable; however, using two of the easier situations will be a disadvantage because it will not provide the extra preparation for facing the more powerful fears.

2. Your child will need your help with identifying the thinking errors and with developing replacement thoughts. Reviewing all of the thinking errors with him will be beneficial and will help both of you to become more familiar with the different types. I also suggest that you highlight (with a highlighter) your child's most common thinking errors in his book. It also is recommended that you share some of your own personal examples of times that you have made thinking errors (if you have a hard time doing this, ask your child which thinking errors he or she thinks you most often make; you may be quite surprised to see how observant your child is when it comes to you!).

Identify and Replace Thinking Errors

Your exercise this week includes:

1. Listing two of your anxiety situations from your ladder and the anxious thoughts you have about these situations.

2. Labeling your thinking mistakes if there are any.

3. Changing your thoughts by creating "replacement thoughts," using the tool below. Remember: Replacement thoughts are balanced and neutral thoughts that do not cause anxiety. (*Hint*: You will know that you came up with a good replacement thought when the thought makes

you feel calmer and more prepared to cope with the scary situation.)

4. Make 10 cards for detached mindfulness. Write down 10 different thoughts (seven, which are typical, neutral thoughts; two of which are anxious thoughts; and one untrue thought). Mix them up and read them three times in a row quickly each day. After reading them, each time say aloud, "I can see these are just thoughts. Whether they are true or not, neutral or scary, they are just thoughts. Thoughts do not have any power unless I give them power." Do this for 2–3 weeks (it shouldn't take more than 3 minutes a day).

EXERCISE

Situation →	Thoughts →	Thinking Error(s)
Replacement Thoughts:		

Situation →	Thoughts →	Thinking Error(s)
Replacement Thoughts:		

EXERCISE

Situation →	Thoughts →	Thinking Error(s)

Replacement Thoughts:

Situation →	Thoughts →	Thinking Error(s)

Replacement Thoughts:

Write your 10 thoughts for Detached Mindfulness practice here:

CHAPTER

6

Changing Your Behaviors

Facing Your Fears

To deal with her anxiety, Kimberly was skilled at avoiding certain situations, such as not being the first to walk into her house. She also regularly sought reassurance from her parents, would throw a tantrum when unexpected changes in the schedule occurred, and she scanned her environment at home for trouble, such as signs of a break-in or ways her dog could get loose. Kimberly and her parents identified these behaviors as anxious behaviors. She then systematically, by taking one step at a time, began to face her fears and gradually became more comfortable doing those things she avoided. When Kimberly asked for reassurance, her parents reminded her that they could not let the anxiety win by giving into it; if she asked if the dog was OK, her mom replied, "Kim, that's the anxiety talking. If I answer you, the anxiety will get stronger and win, and I can't do that as a member of your team." Kimberly sometimes got upset when her mom wouldn't answer, but deep down she knew her mom was right not to listen to the anxiety.

T HIS chapter focuses on preparing your child to face her fears. By now, you and your child have learned about the body and thoughts parts of anxiety; this chapter is on the third part: behavior.

Chapter 5 illustrated how thoughts influence feelings and actions (behavior). Therefore, if your child *feels* afraid of something, she will probably try to avoid it. Children demonstrate other nervous behaviors when they are anxious, including but not limited to the following:

- ▶ reassurance seeking (asking you or another adult for validation or affirmation that a situation is safe and that they are OK);
- ▶ asking a lot of questions (seeking predictability);
- ▶ overplanning activities;
- ▶ repeating information or previously answered questions;
- ▶ clinging (staying near you or another adult);
- ▶ crying;
- ▶ picking (nails, hair, feet, lips, or any other part of one's body);
- ▶ fidgeting;
- ▶ freezing;
- ▶ having a tantrum or meltdown;
- ▶ scanning their environment (looking around for signs that make them feel more relaxed); and
- ▶ rituals (repetitive behaviors typically done to reduce anxiety).

As previously explained, avoidance behavior reinforces anxiety about the situation. To overcome your child's anxiety, you and your child cannot engage in avoidance behavior anymore. I say "you" because most warm and caring parents end up enabling their child to avoid her fearful situations. This is referred to as *accommodation*; you are accommodating her fears to prevent her from having a negative emotional experience. As mentioned in Chapter 2, accommodating your child's anxiety and providing reassurance are common acts of loving, caring parents; however, this behavior is counterproductive as it prevents your child from facing of her fears and confirms for her that the situation she dreads is worth fearing.

Remind your child of the "you against the fear" mindset and encourage her to take a positive attitude. Tell her that she can do this and that she will win! In review, your child will begin at the bottom of her ladder (hierarchy) and will gradually move up, going from least to most anxiety-provoking. Occasionally, children do not accurately rank their fears or an opportunity to do one of the steps presents itself (i.e., they get invited to a sleepover and this is one of their steps), and the two of you will decide to deviate from the order and structure of the ladder. This is perfectly fine, as long as she is OK with doing this. In general, it's really not about feeling "ready" to face your fears; rather, she just needs to do it in order to discover that she can handle it. Most of the time, she will realize that it's not as bad as she originally anticipated it would be. With repetition, she will habituate to the scary situation, making it no longer anxiety-provoking. So, being "ready" is actually more about deciding to do it and to deal with the anxiety that comes up when she faces her fears. It's about being willing to tolerate the discomfort and negative emotions until they dissolve (which will happen once the situation is experienced repeatedly).

Each step on the ladder is called an *exposure*, because your child is being exposed to the anxiety-provoking situation. It is imperative that your child not be forced to do the exposures. Although you can provide encouragement, and maybe even push a little, if you force her to do an exposure, her anxiety may be unintentionally strengthened. If getting your child to cooperate with facing her fears is challenging, refer to Chapter 9, which focuses on motivating your child. If your child is still not cooperative, it may be that the first step is too difficult for her to start with and you may need to help her come up with an easier step, or break the step down into much smaller parts. In fact, breaking the steps into smaller parts or making them "time-limited" (start with doing it for 1 minute) is a good idea for many children, as it makes the task more manageable. Any step can be broken down into smaller steps; whatever is needed to get her moving in the progression of facing her fears. Usually, once children begin to face their fears and have success in doing so, it becomes much easier to get them to face the rest of their fears on the ladder.

Also, I have shared the following good news with your child in his book:

> Once you are done facing all of your fears, there will be a celebration in your honor. You and your parent(s) are going to have a little party to celebrate you and all of your hard work. You may even get an award or a special treat! You might decide to invite a sibling if you have one or a best friend or grandparent to celebrate you with you and your parent.

Remind your child that he is prepared to handle facing his fears and the feelings of anxiety that may arise during the process, even if he doesn't "feel ready." He has tools and strategies for coping and also has your support. The goal is to tolerate the discomfort and get through it. Your child needs to go through facing his fears to get over his fears; he needs to go through the uncomfortable moments. There is no way out but through (and this, by the way, is how kids become resilient). Acceptance and commitment therapy (ACT), which has similarities to CBT, accurately refers to avoidance behavior as "experiential avoidance," because the difficulties lie in experiencing the negative emotions. When these emotions are tolerated, the child learns that it's manageable, that the situation is not that bad, and then the emotions dissolve as she stays in the situation long enough. Then she is the on the path to becoming free from her anxiety.

As he faces his fears, make sure to give a lot of praise and positively reinforce his effort and successes. In addition, encourage him to praise and compliment his success. You and your child together should place the stickers on his hierarchy for each step that he has completed (make sure he is awarding stickers accurately).

The exercise this week is designed to help your child review the strategies he has learned to help manage or cope with his anxiety. It is normal for him to experience anxiety as he begins to face his fears. The goal isn't to not have anxiety; the goal is to cope with it. After all, if it didn't cause him anxiety, it wouldn't be on the ladder. Most children will find that after some initial anxiety, their anxiety significantly decreases as they continue to stick with the exposures. Ultimately, he will experience no anxiety, as he will become desensitized and habituated. I explained to your child in his book that the children I work with always feel great after they face their fears and often report how surprised they were to find that the exposures were not as terrifying as they had expected. This realization also will help motivate your child to continue to face his more challenging fears listed at the top part of his ladder.

You and your child will create a *plan for coping* to prepare him for the exposures. You may need to review this plan several times with him, especially in the beginning; however, if it becomes so repetitive that it resembles reassurance seeking, I recommend that you ask *him* to tell *you* the plan. A plan for coping with the exposures will increase his sense of preparation.

Plan for Coping

A plan for coping will consistently include using the strategies or tools in your child's toolbox that will help him deal with his anxiety when facing his fears. The tools your child has learned in the previous chapters include:

▶ calm breathing;
▶ one-nostril breathing;
▶ progressive muscle relaxation;
▶ relaxing imagery;
▶ asking two important questions;
▶ using positive self-talk (read the cards);
▶ talking back to the anxiety;
▶ dealing with anticipatory anxiety;

- ▶ changing your thoughts (identifying and replacing thinking errors as they come up); and
- ▶ seeing the thoughts as just thoughts and being an observer of the thoughts (detached mindfulness).

Most likely, your child won't use *every* tool in *his* toolbox, just his favorites and most effective ones. Plus, he will likely use different tools for different situations. For example, James (the boy who had a snake phobia) used calm breathing as he looked at pictures of snakes in a book, but he used positive self-talk when he stood near a live snake and challenged his automatic catastrophizing thoughts.

When doing the exposures, you may find that your child becomes so anxious and panicked that he is unable to effectively use the strategies like conquering worry and changing his thoughts. If this happens, encourage him to use distraction techniques in addition to calm breathing to calm down enough to be able to conquer worries and change his thoughts. Examples of distraction techniques include:

- ▶ Make lists using the ABCs: Go through the alphabet and try to come up with lists alphabetically. For example, girls' names (Aileen, Bonnie, Camryn, Denise, Emily, Frances); cities/states/countries (Alabama, Baltimore, Cuba, Delaware, Ecuador, Florida); jobs (artist, baker, chemist, dentist, engineer, firefighter). It can be any topic and if the alphabetizing part is too challenging, you can do the lists without doing them in alphabetical order. This will help distract her from the anxiety-provoking situation.
- ▶ Focusing: Your child can focus on something that she can see (e.g., a tree, book, sneakers) and try to think of five or more different parts of it or ways to describe it (e.g., What color is it? What shape is it? What does it smell like? What does it sound like? What does it feel like? What could you use it for?).
- ▶ Pick a color and think of five things that come in that color.

- ▶ List five favorite books, five favorite songs, or five favorite movies.
- ▶ Counting: Your child could count backward from 100 by 7 (e.g., 100, 93, 86, 79, . . .) or any other number.

Another part of making a plan for coping during exposures is to decide in advance that he will break down the exposure into even smaller steps, as mentioned above. For instance, when James did his first exposure (talking about snakes) he began by talking about snakes for 1 minute, then did it again the next day for 5 minutes, then did it again on the third day for 10 minutes.

When facing fears, review what your plan will involve with your child: Think about which tools he will use and which distraction technique he will rely on if using the tools becomes difficult to accomplish.

When it comes time for your child to do an exposure, he should rate his anxiety on a scale from 0–10. He can rate his anxiety level on a "FEAR-mometer" scale.

    0 = no fear at all/completely relaxed like in a deep sleep

    5 = nervous and scared but not too terrible

  10 = extremely afraid, totally anxious, and panicked

It is essential that when your child is doing the exposures, that *you,* the parent, remain as calm as possible. If he detects that you are anxious, he may feel that there is good reason to feel anxious and have trouble calming down. Be calm and be very encouraging. Display confidence in your child and praise him for each step taken toward facing his fears. Even though in the majority of cases, the child is not forced to face his fears, sometimes it is necessary (e.g., the child who is at risk of not being allowed to go to school due to not being vaccinated would be forced to face his fear of shots/injections). The good news is that even in these cases, the child ends up benefitting from having faced his fears.

Chapter 6 EXERCISE

EXERCISE (sidebar)

Tips for Parents

1. When your child is writing the tools in his toolbox, make sure that he has included most of the tools listed on pages 111–112. When noting his fear level, you can do this verbally, "On a scale from 0–10, where was your anxiety?" Alternatively, you and your child can draw a picture of the FEAR-mometer and he can write in the exposure at the point on the ladder that represents his anxiety level. It also is important for your child to note the changes in his anxiety level (from 0–10) as he stays in the anxiety-provoking situation (e.g., he may start out with an "8" but after 5 minutes he may be down to a "4") and also as he continues to do the same exposure on different occasions (e.g., the first time James looked at pictures of snakes he rated his fear at a "6" but by the fourth time, he rated it as a "1 or 2" because he became used to looking at pictures of snakes).

2. After each exposure, remind your child of his change in anxiety level (e.g., "You did a great job, and your anxiety went down from an 8 to a 4"). The goal is for your child to do each exposure repeatedly—not just once or twice. Ultimately, we want the exposure to cause your child no anxiety, and this will be accomplished with practice, repetition, and prolonged exposure. The three keys of exposure are: **repetition** (do the same situation over and over), **frequency** (practice the situation often, daily if possible; for example, don't wait 6 weeks between sleepovers if that is a step on the ladder), and **prolonged** exposure (stay in the situation long enough for habituation to occur; if going in a room alone is on the ladder, the child should not run in and out of a room for 30 seconds; rather, she should gradu-

ally stay in the room alone for longer and longer stretches of time until she is comfortable being in a room alone).

3. Generally, your child will earn two stars for each exposure (each placed on one side of the ladder for that particular step). The first star will be earned after your child does the exposure for the first time. The second star will be given once your child has practiced the exposure several times and the situation no longer evokes a sense of anxiety. The second star symbolizes that your child has overcome that particular fear or anxiety.

EXERCISE

Facing Your Fears

Your exercise this week includes:

1. Drawing a picture of a toolbox and writing the different "tools" you can use to control your anxiety in your toolbox. (Remember, the tools are the different strategies you can use to manage your anxiety; they are all listed earlier in this chapter.)
2. Taking the first step of your ladder (do your first exposure).
   a. Remember to put stickers on your ladder after you have practiced your first step several times!
   b. Remember to note what your anxiety level was on the FEAR-mometer.

Make your picture of the toolbox look something like this one:

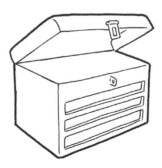

7

Keep Facing Your Fears and Build Confidence

After taking the first step on her ladder—only checking on her dog twice a day— Kimberly was ready to take the next step. Although it was a challenge for her to hold back her urge to check, she relied on her coping plan to help her deal with the exposure. Kimberly used calm breathing, positive self-talk, and distraction to cope with her feelings of anxiety. The longer she went without checking, the easier it was to not check. Kimberly then took her next step on the ladder: doing homework while staying calm. She developed a system of writing down her assignments in checklist form and estimating how long each one would take. She checked off the completed assignments as she went along, reassuring herself that she could handle it and would only focus on the one task at hand. If she noticed that her body felt tense, she stopped for 5 minutes to do calm breathing. With practice, Kimberly learned to be calm when doing her daily homework. Her parents were very supportive and cheered her on, complimenting her for earning stars on her ladder!

THIS chapter also is on the behavior part of anxiety. If you are reading this chapter, it most likely means that your child has faced his or her first fear, so let me officially congratulate you for being so effective in helping your child overcome his anxiety! Taking the first step is a big step for your child, and you should feel very proud of him for getting this far. You also should feel proud of yourself for helping your child get here.

As you can probably predict, the goal at this point is for your child to continue to take the rest of the steps on the ladder one at a time, and the exercise at the end of this chapter is focused on preparing your child to accomplish this. (Remember that Chapter 9 provides guidance on how to motivate your child to complete this program, including how to help her face her fears.) Once all of the steps are taken on the ladder, your child can go on to Chapter 8 (which is the last chapter in her book) and celebrate her success!

Remind your child that while facing her fears is difficult to do, she will feel much better as a result, and also will gain freedom from her anxiety! Soon her anxiety will not dictate how she will feel or think or act. In addition, by facing her fears, your child will feel much better about herself and her self-confidence will strengthen and improve.

It is essential that you encourage your child to feel proud of herself, as this is an indication of healthy self-esteem. Self-esteem develops, in part, when children gain mastery in a certain area, including facing their fears. Keeping in mind that anxiety breeds self-doubt, which may weaken or threaten self-esteem, overcoming anxiety can be an incredibly powerful boost to your child's confidence in himself and can lead to that sense of mastery. Facing one's fears breeds self-confidence. I strongly encourage you to incorporate this aspect into your child's process of overcoming his anxieties and fears. The goal of this book is for your child to master facing his fears.

Self-esteem is also impacted by how a child interprets the events in his life. If he interprets facing his fears as "I should've been able to do this all along," his interpretation is not fostering his self-esteem. Rather, he should acknowledge his accomplishments, or at minimum, should acknowledge the effort that led to them. How he thinks about effort and mastery relates to his "mindset." In the book *Mindset: The New Psychology of Success*, Dr. Carol Dweck (2006) explained that there are two types of mindset: the "fixed mindset," in which the child believes that she is either naturally good at something or she's not, that people are born with a predetermined amount of intelligence, skill, or talent; and the "growth mindset," which views intelligence, skill, and talent as something that can be acquired with effort. In the growth mindset, failure and effort are understood as ways to become smarter, more capable, and so on. Children with the growth mindset are more likely to rise to a challenge and think positively about themselves for putting forth the effort. They also persevere more. When it comes to anxiety and facing one's fears, if your child believes that she is limited and cannot do it, then you should have the discussion of "mindset" with her. If she doesn't celebrate her effort, she may need to practice adopting a growth mindset.

A parent's role in the development of his child's self-esteem is profound. Self-esteem is one of the strongest predictors of success and happiness in adulthood, and I would argue it is far more important than the type of school or college your child will attend. Praising your child is important, but only when it's authentic and either way, overpraise (too much praise and praise for unimportant events) may be counterproductive, as it may cause children to question the authenticity of deserving praise. Ideally, you want it to be a balance between how you celebrate children (external reward) to how they are aware of and feel good about what they are able to do (internal reward). In addition, you can encourage a growth mindset, not by reinforcing that they are "smart" (which implies something you're born with), but instead that they "worked hard and didn't give up." If there is a good grade, a comment such as "Wow, you must have really worked hard. Great job" is better than "You are so smart at math." You can praise your child for being smart, but make sure he knows that the smarts came from working hard and putting forth consistent effort.

Your child will learn the following about self-esteem:

Self-esteem refers to how you feel about yourself, it can be positive or negative. Kids with good self-esteem mostly feel good about who they are and feel proud of their accomplishments. They know that while it feels good for others to think positively about them, that it has to come from the inside, too.

The way you think has a lot to do with your self-esteem. For example, kids who believe that if they work hard and stick with a challenging task, then they will learn more or get better at doing it end up feeling better about themselves in the end. The opposite would be thinking that it doesn't matter how hard you try, you won't get better at it. Kids who know that they can do something to change a difficult situation also have more confidence. The opposite would be feeling that there is nothing you can do. You can *always* do something to change an unpleasant situation, even if it's just changing how you feel about it.

Most kids have trouble with friends at some point when growing up, and this can impact self-esteem. When other kids are mean or tease you, you have to be "assertive" and stick up for yourself. Ignoring doesn't work and actually lets the other kid feel more powerful. It is normal for kids to try to have what's called *social power*. When someone is bossy with you or teases you, they are trying to have power over you. If you don't stick up for yourself, it gives them the power they want. Sticking up for yourself doesn't mean that you have to be aggressive or mean, it just means that you have to talk back to them and show them that they are not making you feel upset (of course, you will be upset and you can tell your friends or family, but not the kid who is teasing you). When you "talk back," you don't want to *ask* them to stop talking to you like that; rather, you want to *tell* them that they cannot talk to you like that. If the same kid is being rude or hurtful to you, you should role-play with your parent what you can say back.

Finally, kids who are *proactive* and make decisions based on their values (what is important to them) feel better about themselves than kids who are *reactive* and make decisions based on how they feel. For example, if you don't feel like doing homework and decided not to do it, then you are being reactive. But if you don't feel like doing homework but value going to school the next day prepared, being respectful to your teachers, and being responsible, then you will do your homework. Being proactive makes life a lot cleaner! By facing your fears, you are learning to not be reactive (which leads to avoidance), but to be proactive and let your values guide you!

When facing her fears, it is very important that your child cheer herself on and encourage herself to do the very thing she is afraid of. Boost her with encouraging comments: "I know you can do this," "You will succeed," "You will earn your stickers," "Remember that you can handle this, and it might not be as bad as you think it will be," and "I believe in you, and you will win!" Once your child succeeds, help her recognize and appreciate her success.

As her parent, it is essential that you start to change the way your respond to her anxiety. As stated, warm and loving parents end up accommodating anxiety, which only makes things worse (it doesn't work, it makes anxiety stronger). The goal is to change what you say in response to her anxiety and attempts to seek reassurance. I list specific examples of what to say in Chapter 12, but the general idea is that instead of answering her with reassurance that everything will be OK, you want to prompt her to challenge her anxiety and anxious thoughts; for example, you may respond with, "I see that you are anxious right now. What can you do to talk back to the anxiety?" By being consistent in responding this way, you will be supporting her efforts to overcome anxiety.

When facing her fears, guide her to follow the order of her ladder. Sometimes children may skip around and this is perfectly fine, as long as your child feels ready for it. The main thing to avoid is pushing your child to do items higher on the ladder before she gets there. Sometimes children realize that they did not order their steps correctly, or they may feel differently about the situations after reading the first six chapters of their book; in either of these cases, skipping around may be appropriate. It is also good to add more steps if you and your child become aware of additional avoidance behaviors to challenge (this often happens once you start facing your fears). In addition, if an opportunity to do one of her steps arises (e.g., she is invited to a sleepover or a birthday party, or it's time to register for summer camp), your child might want to take advantage of the chance to take these steps, even if it requires her to go out of order on her ladder. Again, the primary consideration is that your child is willing to take these steps. Feeling ready, as explained, does not mean that she feels no anxiety about doing it, but instead means that she is willing to try, and perhaps can imagine being able to do it. For the majority of children, once they begin the process of taking the steps and facing their fears, they will have an easier time doing the rest of the steps. Usually, motivating your child in the beginning will be your biggest challenge.

This also is the appropriate time to work with your child on getting rid of his nervous behaviors, as discussed in Chapter 6. Your child most likely has been doing these nervous behaviors for quite some time and thus, you have been used to dealing with them and responding to them for quite some time. The behaviors have been reinforcing for your child, as they have likely provided some (temporary) relief to his anxiety. For example, clinging to you or getting reassurance that it will all be OK has made your child feel more safe and secure, but these behaviors work to strengthen your child's overall anxiety. The best approach to helping your child stop these behaviors is a gradual one, similar to the idea of taking one step at a time on the ladder. Once your child has accomplished three or four steps, it is a good time to introduce the goal of gradually stopping the nervous behaviors. As the parent, you likely will be the one to initiate this process, and your child will benefit from your emotional support as she begins to end this unproductive pattern of coping. Although you can reassure your child that he is capable of stopping and replacing these nervous behaviors, you cannot continue to reassure him in response to his anxiety-driven requests (again, Chapter 12 provides more specific guidance on this).

The first step in helping your child get rid of these behaviors is to point out when they are happening: Help your child become aware of when she is engaging in these behaviors. Label the behaviors as part of the anxiety. In your child's book, he will learn that you will eventually stop giving him the reassurance he seeks and that you are not doing this to upset or punish him. Remind him that providing the reassurance only serves to validate and strengthen the anxiety. Instead, as the parent, you will encourage your child to use his self-talk and relaxation skills to *help himself* feel better.

One option to help modify these nervous behaviors is to use a calendar to track each day that your child does not exhibit the nervous behaviors. For example, before bed, Billy repeatedly asked his mom if he could stay home from school the next day; sometimes she would give in and let him. After coming to therapy, Billy's mom learned that letting him stay home from school was actually making his anxiety worse. His mother then learned to change the way she responded to Billy, and instead she would say, "You sound nervous about going to school, but you have to go. We cannot allow anxiety to control your life. What can you do to calm down right now?" At first, Billy didn't like this response from his mother, but after a while, he got used to it and began to feel OK. They charted his progress on a calendar: Every night that Billy did not ask his mom if he could stay home from school, he earned a check on his calendar. Gradually, he learned that everything turned out fine, even though his mother did not allow him to stay home from school. Additionally, Billy recognized that he felt more confident because he was able to handle his anxiety and worries on his own. He also found school less stressful because he began attending regularly and was able to stay on top of his schoolwork.

Like Billy, your child can get rid of his nervous behaviors and feel better about himself. I recommend that you make a list of which nervous behaviors you observe your child doing, and then help your child gradually reduce the frequency and intensity of each behavior.

Chapter 7 EXERCISE

Tips for Parents

1. In reference to the rest of the steps on the ladder, it will be extremely beneficial if you and your child can generate additional "replacement thoughts" for as many of the remaining anxiety-provoking situations on the ladder. Try to identify the thinking errors that your child is using that maintain his fear of the situation, then come up with a new, more balanced thought. It is not necessary to do this for each and every step on the ladder; however, at minimum, it should be done for the hardest steps and/or the ones that your child is most resistant to facing. Remind you child that we can change the way we think to change the way we feel. The exercise at the end of this chapter includes a chart that you and your child can use to develop replacement thoughts for the different anxiety-provoking situations.

2. You and your child should look at his toolbox before the exposures as a review of what he can do to cope with the anxiety that may arise in the process.

3. If your child struggles to complete a certain step, you may want to break the step down into even smaller steps to make it more manageable. For example, if your child has separation anxiety, one of his steps might be to go to the bathroom alone while you sit outside the door with the door open. Then the next time, you would sit outside with the door closed. In other words, you are helping him create smaller goals to work toward completing the step. It is best to define progress as any movement, no matter how small or gradual, toward the goal. Behavior change usually happens in small steps. Another example would be if your child has social anxiety and one of her steps includes going to a birthday party without you. You can break this down into

smaller steps, starting with walking her in and then leaving after 30 minutes, then leaving after 15 minutes, and then just dropping her off. These types of accommodations are appropriate to use during the exposure phase, and there is a time-limited nature to offering these accommodations; most importantly, they are offered solely for the purpose of helping your child complete the steps, which are a necessary part of the treatment process.

4. Another option is to make additional worry recordings specific for certain steps that are difficult. For example, the child with social anxiety who is afraid of going to the birthday party without a parent can make a recording (if she hasn't already) for the worries specific to the party and the recording can be both a typical worry loop and also uncertainty training (example of recording: "What if no one talks to me? What if the kids are mean? What if I want to leave and no one will get me? I might start crying and then kids will laugh at me. It is always possible that no one will talk to me. It's possible that the kids will be very mean and that I'll want to leave and no one will get me. It's possible that I will start to cry and the kids will laugh at me"). The repetition of worries within the worry tape is good, and framing the worries in both "what if" form and "it is always possible" (uncertainty training) form is ideal.

5. It is normal for children to feel anxious and scared the first couple of times they do a step on their ladder, but you can assure them that it will get easier with practice. This type of assurance is appropriate because it is done in support of the exposure process. In contrast, many children find that they are not anxious or scared at all when they take one of their steps, and when this happens, it is advantageous to help them understand that the anxiety they felt before they practiced was nothing more than anticipatory anxiety.

EXERCISE

This anxious feeling was not a good predictor of the actual experience.

6. One final important note about completing the rest of the steps on your ladder: As a reminder, the goal is for your child to **repeat** each step on his ladder *multiple times*. Children don't just do a step once or twice and then forget about it. Instead, they continue to do it over and over until it no longer makes them feel anxious or scared, with the goal of the behavior becoming integrated into their normal repertoire of behaviors. This also will help to expand your child's comfort zone. So, once your child does something on her ladder, she will continue to do it repeatedly and then it will become something that she is able to do comfortably. It is ideal to have the practices occur as frequently as possible. Finally, it is best if the exposures are prolonged; the longer she stays in the situation, the better (remember the three keys of exposures: repetition, frequency, prolonged).

Good luck with helping your child on the rest of the steps!

Finish Your Ladder

1. Remember to go at your own pace, but try to do 1–2 steps each week. If any step feels like it's too much, try breaking it down into smaller steps. Also, you can make additional worry tapes that are specific for certain steps on your ladder.

2. Don't forget to:
    a. put stickers on your ladder next to the step after you've taken it, and
    b. note what your anxiety level was on the FEAR-mometer.

3. Change the way you think to change the way you feel! Use steps from your ladder for the situation and write down the automatic thought or worry you have about facing that

fear. Then, figure out which thinking error you might have used, and come up with a new, more balanced and accurate thought for your replacement thought. Your parents can help you come up with these new thoughts. When you take each step, try to remind yourself of the replacement thought you came up with for that situation. Good luck!

EXERCISE

Situation →	Thoughts →	Thinking Error(s)
Replacement Thoughts:		

Situation →	Thoughts →	Thinking Error(s)
Replacement Thoughts:		

EXERCISE

Situation →	Thoughts →	Thinking Error(s)

Replacement Thoughts:

Situation →	Thoughts →	Thinking Error(s)

Replacement Thoughts:

8

Lessons Learned

Celebrate Yourself

With dedication and her parents' support, Kimberly successfully faced all of her fears. She practiced having unexpected changes in the schedule, and when it came time for her next dentist appointment, Kimberly's mother deliberately did not tell her until she picked her up from school. Unlike the last time, Kimberly was able to handle it, and she went to the appointment without preparation. She knew that by doing so, she was not letting anxiety rule her life. Kimberly also got used to being the first one to walk into the house, and her heartbeat no longer increased as she did so. She stopped checking on her dog, and homework was a much more pleasant experience. Kimberly and her parents celebrated her great achievement: She completed her ladder and gained freedom from anxiety. There were some bumps in the road along the way, but Kimberly persevered, and overcame her fears. Kimberly and her parents celebrated with a special dinner at her favorite pizza place in her honor. At dinner, her parents shared how proud they were of all of her hard work and great success!

WELCOME to the last chapter of your child's book. Making it here is a tremendous accomplishment and both you and your child deserve a huge "Congratulations!" In honor of completing this program, you will throw a little party (or the like) to celebrate all of your child's hard work and success, and you will present him with the official Certificate of Achievement (located on p. 88 in your child's book). Your child has the option of decorating the certificate, but I recommend that you fill in the lines with your child's name and date and sign it. For the celebration, you and your child can invite other family members like siblings and grandparents, or you can keep it to just the two (or three if his other parent is included) of you. Some children like to have a party at home or prefer to do something else as their celebration, like going to a favorite place or favorite restaurant or doing a special activity. The celebration can be whatever you and your child decide upon; the only requirement is that it is in your child's honor. The party/celebration is a great time to further compliment your child for his excellent participation in this program and help him become aware of the mastery he has gained in the process.

Before the celebration, there are two final areas to address:

1. What lessons did you and your child learn?
2. How can your child handle anxiety and worries if they come up again in the future?

Lessons Learned

Let's review what your child did to get to the point of facing his fears and overcoming his anxiety.

First, your child learned about the three parts of anxiety: body, thoughts, and behavior. After creating his team and team goals and making the ladder, he learned how to work on each of the three parts in order to overcome his anxiety. To address the physiological component of anxiety, your child learned and practiced:

1. calm breathing,
2. progressive muscle relaxation,
3. relaxing imagery,
4. mindfulness meditation, and
5. yoga.

To help with his anxious thoughts, he learned:

1. how to master his worries (worry tapes, uncertainty training);

2. how to use self-talk;
3. about the situation-thought-feeling connection (how you think will affect how you feel, so changing your thoughts can change the way you feel); and
4. about thinking errors and how to change them to healthy replacement thoughts.

Finally, to help with the behavioral component, your child learned how to face her fears, one by one, and she did so by completing the steps on her ladder. She also learned how to get rid of other anxious behaviors and practiced eliminating those as well. Most importantly, your child learned that changing the way she thinks not only changed the way she feels, but it also changed the way she behaved!

By facing his fears, your child learned that he could beat anxiety and overcome it. Children who successfully face their fears also tend to realize that their fears were not as terrible as they anticipated that they would be. Thus, when they were in the different anxiety-provoking situations, they discovered that it was not that bad after all. They stayed with the situation and did not engage in avoidance behavior, and then became used to it; they were able to tolerate feared situations without being afraid.

Your child also learned that when presented with a challenge or obstacle, she can face it and become stronger as a result. Most children experience an improvement in their self-confidence from facing their fears and overcoming anxiety. In this way, they took back the control in their life and became free from the constraints of anxiety-avoidance behavior.

As a parent, you learned not to reinforce your child's fears by accommodating the anxiety. You learned that accommodating the anxiety made it worse, and you challenged your child (and yourself) by not giving in and by remaining firm. In this way, you were an instrumental part of your child's treatment plan. Without your willpower and insights, your child would not have been able to successfully overcome his anxiety.

Handling Worry and Anxiety in the Future (Relapse Prevention)

The majority of children who successfully learn the skills related to understanding and overcoming their anxiety and face their fears do not return to the state of anxiety that they were in at the onset of treatment. In other words, most children do not return to being as anxious as they were when they started the program. However, some children do have relapses (most of the time, these relapses are relatively small and easily worked through). The best part is, if this happens, you and your child know exactly what to do (this is the advantage of CBT)! Your child can handle any future anxiety in the same manner as she did throughout this program. You and your child now have the skills to deal with any anxiety. These skills are yours and can be used at any point in the future.

The following is an example given in your child's book:

James successfully overcame his fear of snakes by completing this program. More than a year went by without thinking about or worrying about snakes when James went to a birthday party and there was a snake trainer there to put on a show (can you believe it?). Because he had not thought about snakes for so long, when he first saw the huge snake around the neck of the trainer, James suddenly felt a rush of fear. For a moment, he forgot that he was no longer scared of snakes! Then he realized that he knew what to do: He knew that he needed to stay at the party, and actually sat closer to the snake trainer to make it more like he was facing his fears. He also took a few deep breaths and remembered that he could handle this. He reminded himself that he would be OK and that he's done this before so he can do it now. After about 5 minutes, James felt back to normal again. He was calm and felt no fear. James was reminded that whenever he felt anxious, he just needed to use the tools in his toolbox and face his fears. Like James, you may have some anxiety and worry from time to time. Just do what you have throughout this program, and you'll be fine. Keep this book someplace safe and come back to it whenever you need to. I know that everything will work out for you, and I wish you all the best in your future.

The key to preventing relapse is to encourage your child to face any fears that may arise in the future. As soon as you observe any avoidance behavior, try to nip it in the bud by having your child face his fears. Some children have returned for tune-up appointments and some present with a few (and often new) anxieties or fears. For these children, I often will make another "mini-ladder," with three to five steps on it to address the anxiety-provoking situations, and will have them review their self-talk note cards and other exercises (at the end of each chapter). New worry tape recordings can be made as well, if necessary. Because they have successfully completed the treatment and have overcome their past fears, this process is generally very smooth and only takes a short time.

Keep in mind that not all things that your child doesn't want to do is a fear; sometimes it is simply a preference. For example, a girl with social anxiety may prefer to only invite one friend over at a time. Although this could be interpreted as anxiety (e.g., she is afraid if she has more than one friend over, she'll be left out/excluded), it could likely be that she just prefers to invite only one friend rather than inviting more friends over at the same time (enjoys one-on-one time more). Asking your child for clarification, "Is this something that makes you feel uncomfortable or nervous, or this is something you like better?" and scanning for visible signs of anxiety are the best ways to assess the situation. Also, look for signs of anxiety, such as what the child says about the event (e.g., is he describing worries or concerns about it?) or if he exhibits other nervous behaviors.

Chapter 8 EXERCISE

Tips for Parents

1. The party and receiving the Certificate of Achievement is an important part of your child's participation in the program. The concept of acknowledging and celebrating one's achievements, and feeling positive about accomplishing hard work is an important component for healthy self-esteem development. This is your chance to model this for your child and help your child celebrate herself!

2. The details of the party will be discussed by you and your child. It does not have to involve spending a lot of money; rather, the spirit of the celebration is what counts.

3. Some parents choose to frame their child's certificate after it is completed and/or decorated.

Celebrate Yourself With a Party and Earn Your Official Certificate of Achievement!

1. Talk to your parent about the party and who should come to it. Some kids have the party with just their one or two parents, and others invite their siblings, pets, or friends. There is no right or wrong way to do it—the only rule is that you have fun and celebrate all of your hard work and success!

2. For the Certificate of Achievement, you and your parent can complete the form and you can decorate it anyway you like! Have a great party—you deserve it! I am so proud of you!

9

Motivating
Your Child

MOST parents will benefit from reading this chapter early on in the course of this program. Making the ladder usually motivates the child with anxiety. This chapter offers several different approaches to help motivate your child to read the book, do the exercises, and face her fears. The goal is to be able to complete the program as a self-help resource; however, if after implementing the techniques described in this chapter you are unable to get your child engaged in the process, I recommend that you seek professional help. The Resources for Parents section at the end provides links to finding an appropriate therapist in your area.

It is important that you do not force your child to read the book and/or complete the program, or punish your child for a lack of participation. Always start with empathizing, showing that you understand how hard it is for her and how scary it feels to face the anxiety. But the empathy should be blended with the expectation that the anxiety needs to be treated. You want your child to understand that something needs to be done to address the anxiety, and that this is where you chose to start. You can always offer to break down a step into smaller steps by saying, "What are you willing to do?" but forcing or scolding is not the way to go when it comes to treating childhood anxiety.

Some children with anxiety will also have oppositional defiant disorder (ODD) and throw tantrums, be aggressive, and exhibit defiance when their parents ask them to cooperate; when it is true oppositional defiant behavior, this defiance will show up regularly when the child is *not* anxious or *not* in anxiety-provoking situations (versus the anxious child who will tantrum and throw a fit mostly in response to being in an anxiety-provoking situation or anticipating one). Although every child misbehaves and pushes the limits at times, children with ODD frequently lose their temper, are easily annoyed and set off, blame others for their misbehavior, and are disrespectful to parents and often teachers/other adults or authority figures; the ODD causes a problem at home and likely at school and socially. If your child has ODD, I recommend that this be addressed first before treating the anxiety. The approach I have found to be most effective is *The Kazdin Method for Parenting the Defiant Child* by Dr. Alan Kazdin (see Resources section).

The ideal age range for *Anxiety-Free Kids* is 7–14. Some of the motivational techniques described in this chapter will be more appropriate for younger children while others will be more appropriate for early teens. Finally, some children will get stuck on not wanting to read the book, and others will show resistance toward doing the exposures. Therefore, this chapter is divided into five sections:

1. general principles of reinforcement,
2. motivational strategies for younger children not willing to read the chapters,
3. motivational strategies for younger children not willing to do the exposures,
4. motivational strategies for early teens not willing to read the chapters, and
5. motivational strategies for early teens not willing to do the exposures.

General Principles of Reinforcement

First, let me clarify that, in general, the treatment of childhood anxiety disorders should not incorporate discipline strategies—this is not a behavioral problem in the classic sense. Rather, childhood anxiety disorders describe a mental condition that often involves a great deal of pain and discomfort. Being punished for not being able to face one's fears only serves to exacerbate this pain and discomfort. Although most children with anxiety disorders have symptoms that are not visible (e.g., internal thoughts, self-talk, self-doubt), some children's anxiety manifests as tantrums and meltdowns. However, these are unlike the tantrums and meltdowns that we often see in children who cannot get their way (or who have oppositional defiant disorder as described above), as the behavior is rooted in a very strong drive to avoid anxiety-provoking situations.

The sections below will provide guidance on how to deal with a child's unwillingness to read the chapters and/or do the exposures. Some children with anxiety disorders are also difficult behaviorally in general (not at the extreme level of ODD) and require a consistent discipline approach to help them become more cooperative. Reward/sticker charts can be used for behaviors that fall outside the scope of anxiety (e.g., getting ready on their own, on time, in the morning, doing homework, following routines).

In general, reinforcement is used to increase the occurrence of a behavior and the behavior we are targeting is participation in this program. Positive reinforcement describes the act of rewarding a child with something desirable once he has done a good job. For example, if your child washes your car and you give your child $5, he is more likely to wash your car again because he enjoyed earning the money. Negative reinforcement describes the act of removing something undesirable once he has done a good job. For example, if your child washes your car and as a result does not have to do any other chores like the laundry or cleaning his room, he is more likely to wash your car again because he avoided doing something that he found unpleasant. Both positive and negative reinforcement are effective strategies for promoting desirable behavior. The use of positive reinforcement, in particular, will help your child be cooperative with this program.

Examples of positive reinforcement include earning stickers or privileges (such as 20 minutes of screen time) for reading chapters and completing the exposures, keeping a chart and checking off the progress, giving your child praise for his cooperation and hard work, and, most importantly, being able to do activities he previously avoided because he is no longer afraid to do them! Negative reinforcement has an important role as well—doing the exposures naturally results in the removal of unpleasant anxiety, and therefore your child will be more motivated to do additional exposures.

Motivational Strategies for Younger Children Not Willing to Read the Chapters

Prior to implementing any of the strategies below, I recommend that you attempt to understand your child's resistance to beginning the program. There are many potential and understandable explanations for his unwillingness to start. For instance, your child may simply be afraid of the idea of change (many anxious children resist change and transitions in general), or he may not be willing to recognize the impairment that results from having the anxiety, or he may not like the idea of having to actually do the work of dealing with the anxiety (think of how many adults resist going to therapy because the thought of addressing their problems seems too daunting!). Try to validate your child's feelings and concerns, then boost him up with encouragement and rational statements such as, "I know the idea of doing this seems like a lot—even overwhelming to you—but your worries (or fears or anxiety) are causing an interference and we need to work together to address them," "I'm going to do my part, too. See, I have my own book that I'll be reading while you read yours," and "We're going to take one chapter at a time, and check it off as we go."

Draw a table similar to that in Table 4 and check it off as it is completed.

Show your child the table and explain that she will earn a check for each chapter she reads and for each exercise she completes. The number of checks earned can equal a privilege, if necessary, a very small reward of some kind (usually this applies to younger children and it can be small, inexpensive prizes typically found in a prize bin like bouncy balls). Once your child gets to Chapters 7 and 8, she will begin earning stars on her ladder, which is incredibly rewarding.

If the checklist and small prizes do not help to motivate your child to read the chapters on his own, you may want to attempt to read your child's book to him. For children with reading disorders or for those who do not like to read, reading to them may be the best option. Give her advance notice that you will help her get started and that the two of you will sit down to read at, for example, 5 p.m. Pick an area of the house that she likes (alternatively, you and your child can go somewhere like a park) and sit down and read to her, suggesting that she help you read some of the chapter, even if it's just a sentence or two. See how it goes; if she quickly becomes open to reading it, you may not need to help her for the remaining chapters; however, if she maintains her disinterest in reading it, I would plan on reading Chapter 2 to her later in the week, then reevaluate.

Occasionally, a child is too young or not at the right point developmentally to be receptive to the program, and in this case, waiting for a period of 6 months to a year then trying again may be beneficial. In my clinical practice, I have occasionally worked with a child who was not initially receptive to treatment, but when they returned about a year later, participation was great and the anxiety was successfully overcome.

Table 4
Checklist

	Read Chapter	Did Exercise
Chapter 1		
Chapter 2		
Chapter 3		
Chapter 4		
Chapter 5		
Chapter 6		
Chapter 7		
Chapter 8		

Finally, if the reward system and reading to your child doesn't work and she continues to refuse to read the book, then I would seek additional support, whether it's from your child's pediatrician, the school counselor, or another mental health professional (see Resources section).

Motivational Strategies for Younger Children Not Willing to Do the Exposures

Many children will have at least some resistance to taking the first step or two on the ladder, so it is best to normalize this for your child. Help her understand that it is normal to feel anxious about taking the first step, yet emphasize that she can handle the feelings of anxiety and now has ways to cope with these feelings and that these feelings generally subside once she is completing her exposures. Emphasize that she now has tools for managing her anxiety and facing her fears.

If your child maintains that she is unwilling to try the first step, engage in a discussion with her and seek to understand the reasons. Is it possible that the first step on the ladder is actually too hard to be a first step? Is there another step that seems easier or can she think of an easier situation that is not listed on the ladder? Alternatively, can the first step be broken down into smaller parts to make the tasks more manageable? The key here is to maintain that complete avoidance is no longer an option—she must be willing to try something—and the fact that you are willing to work with her on what that may be shows that you are offering your support and care about her feelings.

Remind your child that he will earn stars on his ladder when he takes a step. (Refer to Chapter 6 for an explanation on how to award stars or stickers if needed). You can emphasize the opportunity to earn rewards and create the Reward List if you haven't already done so.

Motivational Strategies for Early Teens Not Willing to Read the Chapters

Many teens also will respond to a checklist (by the teen years, rewards shouldn't be used). Some young teens will be embarrassed about the program and therefore will reject it. In this case, I recommend that you help reframe the meaning of this program for your teen. Explain that the author works with adults and takes the same approach with them (including making a ladder); this is how anxiety is best treated. Explain that using this program and learning how to overcome his anxiety is a sign of resourcefulness, which is a strong indication of maturity. Highlight the social benefits to overcoming his anxiety, and speak openly that as his parent, you don't want to see him miss out in life because of untreated anxiety. Also, give him permission to keep the fact that he is doing the program private; it is his choice if he wants to share it with others or not.

I caution parents to be careful not to conceptualize seeking professional help as a punishment in any way; seeking professional help is a form of treatment and something to feel good about; it's never a form of punishment. Yet, for teens with anxiety that causes significant impairment in their life, it is only fair that it is calmly explained to them that their anxiety requires treatment, whether it is in the self-help form of this program or with a weekly meeting with a mental health professional. Explain that you have selected this program for them as a first step, and while it may be enough for them to overcome their anxiety, additional professional support may be warranted even once they have completed it. Try to explain in the most loving and supportive way possible that it's your job as a parent to help them be as healthy as possible, and this includes psychological (or emotional) health.

Motivational Strategies for Early Teens Not Willing to Do the Exposures

As stated above, many children will have at least some hesitation when taking the first step or two on the ladder, so it is best to normalize this for your child. Empathize with your child and explain that it is normal for him to be nervous. The section above, "Motivational Strategies for Younger Children Not Willing to Do the Exposures" applies for teens as well. An additional concern for teens is that they may be more sensitive to the social repercussions of doing exposures. They may be concerned about the fact that they have to do exposures and may feel ashamed about it. In this case, it is helpful to normalize these feelings, yet emphasize that the benefits outweigh the costs. You can normalize his feelings by making comments such as, "It makes sense that this is uncomfortable for you—these are things that you have avoided doing for a long time. Taking these steps is supposed to be hard at first," and "The book says that it is normal to feel nervous when facing your fears and the goal is to manage these feelings. If it wasn't hard, it wouldn't be on the ladder."

Because one of the primary tasks of adolescence is identity development, it is particularly important to help your early teen develop confidence in himself and his ability to overcome anxiety. One way of promoting this process of confidence development is by not accommodating his anxiety (again, this can be accomplished in a gradual manner). Ultimately, this forces your child to deal with the anxiety situation on his own, and this in and of itself will likely serve as a motivator to do the exposures. Once he realizes that you will no longer do the accommodations, he likely will become more motivated to face his fears by doing the exposures. Basically, it can start with change at the family-system level. Let me provide a case example:

> Frank was a very bright and very kind 13-year-old boy with OCD. One of his obsessive thoughts involved not killing insects that were in his house; he insisted that they be saved and brought outside of the house. However, he refused to do this himself, as he feared coming into contact with the insects. For many years, Frank's family accommodated his anxiety by rescuing various insects (spiders, roaches, moths) from their home, despite their own preference for killing them and flushing them down the toilet. During Frank's treatment with me, we constructed a ladder and included a step on saving bugs on his own. Although he initially protested, he realized that his family would no longer be accommodating him in this way. When it came time to take that step, Frank was able to do it. In fact, he did great! He saved bugs without a problem and even grew comfortable with the idea of killing them from time to time (a rather "normal" event, he learned, as some bugs potentially pose a health threat if left to live inside houses). He even reminded his family members that it was up to him to save the bugs. Frank gained confidence in his newfound freedom to take care of the problem on his own, and Frank's

family was grateful to no longer have the responsibility of rescuing bugs found in their house. Frank's identity was now beginning to form out of a sense of confidence and mastery, rather than fear and avoidance.

If you find that no matter what you try, you still cannot get your child to cooperate, you can offer two choices: that he can complete the program with another (adult) family member or seek professional help. But doing nothing is not an option. As mentioned in the Introduction, if you do seek professional help, you can request that the therapist use this program with your child (this will be particularly important if the clinician is not very familiar with CBT).

10

Special Sections

THIS chapter provides additional information and tips on how to help your child depending on which type of anxiety she is experiencing. I recommend reading the section(s) that pertains to your child, as well as the sections at the end on how to handle social situations that are impacted by your child's anxiety (e.g., parties, play dates, explaining the issue to other parents).

Generalized Anxiety Disorder (GAD)

As mentioned in Chapter 1, children with GAD have excessive worry that is difficult to contain. They struggle with "what if . . . " thoughts and with tolerating uncertainty, and this is evidenced by their repetitive questioning of what will happen, what happens if . . . , what the plan will be, how they can be prepared, and so on. Part of overcoming GAD, then, involves helping them deal with not knowing everything that will or might happen. For this reason, worry tape recordings and uncertainty training (described in Chapter 4) are essential for getting children with GAD to overcome their anxiety. By modeling your own tolerance for uncertainty, for example, with comments like "It is always possible that we will be late," and "It is always possible that I might get the flu, too," you show your child that it is OK not to know everything that is to come, and that you are happy even without knowing what might happen in the future.

Encourage your child to practice uncertainty training and give her examples on what she can repeat to herself: "It's always possible that I'll get sick and miss the play. It's always possible I'll throw up." Again, as with worry tape recordings, the goal is for your child to gradually become unalarmed/bored by the anxious thoughts about what might happen. The additional goal is feeling like they can handle what comes their way. We do not always know what will happen in life, and we cannot possibly prepare ourselves for the future; all we can do is assure ourselves that we can handle whatever comes our way (which supports a resilient mindset). It also is a good idea to incorporate exposure to unexpected changes in the schedule into your child's ladder. For instance, you can recommend including on the ladder "last minute change in plans," or "Mom is late when picking up the carpool from school" (arrive 10 minutes late, but your child should not know how late you will be). Alternatively, the step can be "unexpected changes in the plan" and then you can decide last minute to go to a different movie, different restaurant, or have a grandparent drive the carpool for a change. The general idea is for your child to practice things not going exactly as planned, and these opportunities will allow her to realize that unexpected changes are normal and can be tolerated. This way, your child will practice stepping outside of her comfort zone.

Because children with GAD usually catastrophize (i.e., expect the worst, visualize disaster) and have excessive worries, sometimes it is appropriate that you help your child adopt more reality-based thoughts. For example, I worked with an 8-year-old girl who walked by an abandoned gym bag on the sidewalk and worried that "sick germs" could have been in the bag and that when walking by it, she could have caught those germs and gotten sick. I explained to her that bags do not hold sick germs in them and that it is impossible to get sick from walking by a gym bag. This explanation encouraged her to adopt more reality-based patterns of thinking. Although it won't cure the anxiety, children with GAD can benefit from some education about the likelihood of what they worry about actually happening, especially if they integrate these facts into their self-talk process. For example, "I know when I'm worrying that it's only the anxiety talking because you cannot get sick from walking by bags." Children with a fear of flying should be told that "flying is not dangerous" and "there are about 28,000 flights every day in the U.S." and should integrate these facts into their self-talk to use when taking a flight.

Children with GAD often have symptoms of restlessness, difficulty concentrating, sleep disturbance, and irritability. Children with GAD can seem preoccupied and find it difficult to pay attention; in my experience, some children with GAD have been misdiagnosed with Attention Deficit/Hyperactivity Disorder (ADHD). It is imperative that an ADHD diagnosis is made only after a thorough neuropsychological assessment in which a battery of tests has been administered. In addition, true ADHD doesn't usually improve on its own without medication, whereas GAD may fluctuate in its severity. If your child is anxious and inattentive, I recommend treating the anxiety first and then reevaluating the inattentiveness. Keep in mind that it is always possible that a child with ADHD also has GAD or has "learning-disorder induced anxiety" (i.e., anxiety from not being able to complete work on time, getting in trouble in school and at home for not paying attention or properly completing tasks).

Children with GAD tend to have a lower tolerance for stress, and therefore they are more easily overwhelmed. For this reason, children with GAD benefit from practicing relaxation, exercising, and doing yoga. We are not designed to go-go-go and it's important to train your child with GAD to incorporate time every day for self-care and relaxation. Overscheduled children with anxiety often can experience relief when their commitments are reduced.

I strongly believe that children need at least one day of the weekend when they are not doing any homework and can have time to relax. Recreational time is essential for creativity. Similarly, if your child maintains an "I must get all A's" attitude in school, I recommend that "earning a B" on a test or assignment be a step on her ladder. Many children with GAD also are perfectionists and come from high-achievement-oriented families (read the section on perfectionism on page 166). The end goal is to put goals in perspective and ensure that children have time to relax, have downtime, can play outside, and have opportunities to be creative in a natural, unstructured way. Children benefit from playtime and also from having some time to spend alone. The goal is to have a good work-play balance.

Separation Anxiety Disorder (SAD)

Children with SAD can present parents with quite a challenge, as they often display excessive clinginess or neediness. They often have a limited tolerance for being without a parent and will melt down upon separation. Children with SAD typically worry about their parent getting hurt or something bad happening. There are varying degrees of this anxiety: Some children constantly seek physical contact with the parent (e.g., a child may hold tightly to his mother's arm) or have trouble with separation, such as when the parent leaves the house, while others may only have difficulty at bedtime and refuse to sleep alone (for sleep, read Chapter 11). During the beginning of the treatment process, it is important to reassure your child that by learning how to tolerate being separate, he is not going to be less loved by you, nor will your bond be threatened in any way. In fact, parents may feel less annoyed by their child as he becomes less clingy or learns to sleep alone, and this may allow for more enjoyable time together; however, I would not share this information with your child as it may be hurtful to hear. Comments such as, "I love you all the time, whether I'm with you or not," "It is perfectly safe to sleep alone, and I know you will be OK," and "We are always very close in our hearts, and anytime you want to feel my love for you, just look inside your heart" can be grounding for your child and give him extra support during the ladder practices. Eventually, you will not give reassurance but instead will cue your child to use the techniques to manage his anxiety.

When developing the steps on the ladder, it likely will be necessary to offer smaller steps within each step. For example, let's say that one step is "Mom goes out without you." Your child may need to practice this several times, starting with a 15-minute interval, then gradually increasing (e.g., by 30 minutes) until your child can tolerate a 2–3 hour period in which you go out without him. At first, you may make yourself available with a cellular phone, but ultimately your child should be able to do the practice without calling you and this should be clearly stated on the ladder (no calling or texting). It is my assumption that your child is with a trusted adult during these separation practices or is old enough and mature enough to stay at home alone. Your child likely will benefit from the following empathic, supportive statements from you: "I know it feels scary and that you don't like it, but you will learn to feel OK when I go out," "It is important for us to work together to help you feel more comfortable when we're not together," and "I know it might not feel this way now, but you will feel better about yourself once you are able to do this."

Sometimes children develop symptoms of SAD after they have experienced a trauma, such as a loss of a parent, abuse, or witnessing a violent act. Additionally, some adopted children develop SAD in response to the disruption of, or lack of, a primary caregiver. In these cases, it is important to give the child some time to cope with the trauma or adjust to the new adoptive home, before you label it as SAD and treat it. At times, the separation anxiety symptoms are transitory and will resolve on their own as time passes and the child adjusts to the traumatic or stressful situation. However, if symptoms persist after 6–12 months (depending on the event), or if the symptoms worsen in severity, then treatment of the SAD likely is warranted.

Social Anxiety Disorder (Previously called Social Phobia, SoP)

Social anxiety disorder, or social phobia, ranges from mild to severe, and goes beyond discomfort with giving presentations in class, such as oral book reports. Although some children with social anxiety often appear painfully shy and will go to great lengths to avoid social behaviors, such as greeting other children, calling friends, initiating plans, and going to parties, others avoid in subtle ways such as not asserting themselves because they are internally questioning if others like them. There are a few thinking errors that are more common to social anxiety than the other anxiety disorders, including mind reading and personalization. It will be very helpful for you to point out when your child is making these thinking mistakes. These thinking mistakes can be evident in normal conversation, such as "I know that my soccer coach doesn't like me," and "My friend cancelled our plans because she is mad at me for not calling her back the other day." It is recommended that you help your child consider other explanations for her coach's or friend's behavior. Additionally, it is important that you do not model being judgmental of others, as the child with social anxiety will use this as evidence that others are judging her as well. For example, commenting that someone on TV is "nervous and shaky" gives the cue to your child that others may be making negative judgments about her when she gets up in front of an audience to talk (e.g., book report).

Because social anxiety may contribute to low self-esteem, it is recommended that you challenge your child with questions like,

"What would someone who is secure with him- or herself think or do in this situation?" or "How would someone who feels confident about him- or herself handle this?" Challenging thoughts by encouraging your child to consider evidence against her anxious thoughts and predictions is another strategy: "What evidence or proof do you have that this will happen?" Additionally, I recommend that you pay attention to the messages that you give regarding mistakes and failures (see more about this in Chapter 12). It is important to communicate that everyone makes mistakes and that people should be forgiving of themselves when mistakes occur. Similarly, we all do embarrassing things from time to time, and the goal is to foster self-acceptance and forgiveness during these times. Also, children should learn that the cues they give to others regarding their mistakes or embarrassing moments tend to be what others use to know how to respond. For instance, if a child trips and falls in front of others, then gets up and smiles or laughs a bit, others will likely smile or laugh, too.

Many years ago, I was at a wedding and confused a man with the father of the bride; I went on and on complimenting him on the beautiful ceremony, the band, the flowers, how beautiful his daughter looked, and then he corrected me: He wasn't the father of the bride. What an embarrassment! I was so embarrassed and kept playing the scenario over and over in my head, until I finally gave myself a pep talk and told myself that everyone makes mistakes and this was a nice reminder of my human-ness. I also focused on how well this man handled it: For the rest of the evening, he kept joking with me, calling me "Lonnie, I mean Ronnie," instead of "Bonnie." Should a similarly embarrassing moment occur for you, it offers an opportunity to model how well you handled it: Share the story with your son or daughter and use a sense of humor to show him or her that it's not so bad after all.

An important skill for all children, but particularly those with social anxiety, is the skill of assertiveness. Assertiveness, or "sticking up for yourself," differs from aggressiveness as it is respectful of the other person(s) and does not include being physical or forceful. It also differs from being passive (doing nothing) as it is an active behavior. Being assertive is an appropriate, healthy behavior indicative of good self-esteem. When others invade our personal space or discount our personal rights, it is appropriate to respond in an assertive manner. For example, if your child has a friend come over and this friend begins to use her fancy art supplies without asking, it is important that your child be assertive and say, "I'm sorry but you need to ask first before using my paints," or "I am the only one who uses my paints, but I am happy to share my nail polish with you." Although sharing is a positive friendship skill, children also have the right to have their personal space and personal property respected, and it is acceptable to have certain things that are not for sharing. Another example is when your child wants to play with other kids and instead of just joining, they ask to join; *asking* to join is not as assertive and it allows the other children to have the social power (because they can say "no, you can't play with us); rather, you should encourage your child to simply join by saying something like "What are you guys playing?" or just observe and join in the play without commenting.

Because children with social anxiety are oversensitive to being judged negatively by others, they are less likely to be assertive, as it incorporates a social behavior that requires confidence and often social risk (e.g., we do not always get the response we'd like, some may take offense). Thus, overcoming social anxiety requires the development of healthy assertive behavior. Parental modeling is an excellent way of showing children how to be assertive. When coaching your child on how to respond in an assertive way, encourage him to maintain good eye contact, stand straight up (no slouching), use a firm, steady voice (not too loud but not soft either), and speak clearly. Nonverbal communication is key; in fact, a classic UCLA study by Albert Mehrabian (Mehrabian & Ferris, 1967) found that 93% of communication is nonverbal (55% through body language and 38% through tone and inflection of voice), so help your child improve his body language, physical presence, and how his voice sounds when being assertive. Initially, you can have discussions with your child *after* the opportunity to be assertive has presented itself and you and your child can discuss how he could have handled the situation in an assertive way. If your child is open to it, you can practice (role-play) the assertive response.

This book does not address in-depth selective mutism, a severe form of social phobia characterized by a tendency to refuse to speak with certain people while being completely comfortable speaking fluently and naturally with others. The Resources section of this book includes a book on this topic. Finally, it is noted that many children with school refusal/school phobic behavior have an underlying social anxiety disorder. Please see the sections below on selective mutism or school refusal if applicable.

Specific Phobia (SP)

Specific phobias can be categorized as "animal type," "natural environment type," "blood-injection-injury type," "situational type," or "other," (such as situations that may lead to vomiting or characters in costume) and again, are differentiated from "fears" as they either involve avoidance of the situations or the situation is tolerated with extreme distress. Situations that often are avoided or intensely feared are flying on planes, being near dogs, going downstairs by themselves, getting sick, and vomiting. Many of the children that I have worked with have the animal type, as they demonstrate an intense fear of dogs, bugs, snakes, spiders, and so forth. The most important advice I give to parents is to show compassion! Having compassion and empathy for your child, even when you don't and can't "get it," is a tremendous gift that you can give. As the nature of a phobia is usually irrational, and the child's reaction to the feared situation is intense and extreme, it is easy for children to feel shamed by their phobia (particularly when most of the other kids they know are not afraid). To prevent this from happening, you can communicate empathy and compassion with comments such as, "I understand how scary this is for you," "I understand how scared you are," and "I know how hard this is for you."

Many parents tell me that they cannot understand why their child cannot just play with a dog, for example. "I don't know what is so bad about a cute, harmless dog? Couldn't we just have our daughter play with a dog so she could see that it is OK?" Well-intentioned parents who genuinely want their child to get over the fear make these types of comments. I respond by giving them advice on how to foster and demonstrate empathy. What seems easy to you is excruciatingly painful for them. Although this may be hard to imagine, it may help to consider a time when you felt extremely scared or panicked, for example, if you nearly got in an accident or couldn't find your child in a store, and realize that this is likely your dog-phobic child's experience when he sees a dog.

Depending on the type of phobia your child has, giving him facts or other information about the feared situation can be beneficial. For instance, for children who avoid flying on a plane due to fears of crashing, it would be appropriate to share that, on average, 40,000 people die every year in car accidents whereas only 100 or so die in plane accidents. You do not want to make your child afraid of cars (and typically this will not), but illustrate how we are used to and not afraid of things that are done routinely on a regular, daily basis, such as driving. Also, your child should learn that flying is the safest form of travel and that skilled technicians conduct mechanical tests on each plane before it flies, making it very safe. Turbulence poses no threat to aircraft safety and equates to just a few bumps in the road in a car or the water in a boat. A coping plan for flying exposure would include (in addition to relaxation strategies, challenging catastrophic and other thinking errors, and positive self-talk) bringing along a host of distraction activities, such as a book, a deck of cards, a music player, a stuffed animal, and puzzles. Self-talk for flying examples include: "Flying is the safest form of travel," "Turbulence is normal and safe," "Once we take off, I will get used to flying and feel comfortable," and "I have a lot of things that I will do to distract myself. I always feel better when I listen to music." Similarly, children who are afraid of dogs should learn that most dogs are harmless and won't bite, although there are certain techniques to use when approaching a dog, such as asking the owner if the dog is safe to touch, approaching the dog slowly but confidently, putting your hand out in a "fist-bump" posture in front of the dog's mouth/nose which allows him to come to your child first, and letting the dog sniff you first. When treating dog phobias, I work with a dog trainer who brings a variety of dogs, and he teaches the child how to put their knee up in front of them (just lift up one leg, raising the knee high enough until it aligns with the stomach), which gives the dog the message not to jump up on the child (it basically blocks the dog from doing so). Providing this step-by-step structure often is grounding for the child with phobias and offers her a planned out approach to working through the situation.

Obsessive-Compulsive Disorder (OCD)

Obsessive-compulsive disorder is a little different from the other anxiety disorders in childhood, and therefore the treatment varies a bit. In the DSM-V, OCD is in its own category, separated out of the category of anxiety disorders. The DSM-V organized the list of disorders in order of relation, so the category of "Obsessive-Compulsive and Related Disorders" (which includes tics, trichotillomania [hair pulling], body dysmorphic disorder, and hoarding disorder) is placed after the category of "Anxiety Disorders," recognizing that OCD relates to anxiety. OCD can be more subtle than other anxiety disorders. I am always amazed at how hidden the symptoms can be, and many parents echo that amazement. For example, children may walk in a certain way, so as to avoid cracks on the sidewalk or walk in a symmetrical fashion (e.g., left foot first in the first square on the block, then right foot first in the second square, or left side of foot touches rim of square on the sidewalk, then right side of foot touches the opposite rim), or do a variety of subtle behaviors that often are missed by others around them (e.g., flicking their hand in a certain way in response to an unwanted thought). For these reasons, giving your child permission to discuss the rituals and creating an open environment to do so is crucial. I find that children respond when I am confident during the inquiry process, "So, I know bathrooms are hard for you—do you avoid touching the flusher, toilet seat, stall lock, faucet, and bathroom door handle? Is there anything you are able to touch?" I make it known that it is usually pervasive (covers a lot of behaviors in the anxiety situation) and that many rituals are involved in OCD. There can also be mental rituals, such as reviewing images over and over and counting every word they read.

Sometimes children can have a form of OCD in which there are only these mental rituals without explicit or observable behaviors (just a mental experience), and this is referred to as *Pure-O*. In most cases, there often are mental actions or mental compulsions that children do in response to the obsessive thoughts. For example, a client of mine with Pure-O would get mentally stuck on a very specific and irrelevant component of a math equation and in response to the obsessive thoughts about it, she would run through the equation over and over for hours until it "felt right." This goes beyond simply obsessive thinking, is incredibly time-consuming, and results in an impairment of some kind (in this case, difficulty focusing in class or when conversing with others). With Pure-O, the goals are the same as with other types of OCD; the child is exposed to the triggering thoughts or images and learns how to not respond with mental acts or rituals (exposure/response prevention; see below). By deliberately calling up the trigger, the child is facing her fears and learns that overcoming OCD involves her not doing the mental rituals.

Children with OCD often are perfectionistic as well as obsessive-compulsive, and this perfectionism may or may not be part of the OCD. See the section on perfectionism on page 166 for more information. All-or-nothing thinking and catastrophizing also are commonly seen in children with OCD.

There are a few additional thinking errors specific to OCD (explained in the book by Hyman and Pedrick described below, as well as in *Metacognitive Therapy for Anxiety and Depression* by Adrian Wells), including "thought-action fusion," "thought-event fusion," "superstitious thinking," and "magical thinking." The fusion-thoughts are part of "Overimportance of Thoughts," which is when the child gives a lot of power to the thoughts, so the thoughts are experienced more as fact than as thoughts. Depending on your child's age, you may or may not choose to discuss these with him. Listed below are definitions and examples of each:

- ▶ **Thought-Action Fusion:** If I have a thought about or urge to do something, then that means that I will do it.
    a. *Example:* "If I have the urge to start a fire at home, then I better stay away from the kitchen and from matches to make sure I don't do it."
    b. *Example:* "If I think about hurting my brother then it means I'm going to do it, so I better not be alone with him."

- ▶ **Thought-Event Fusion:** If I have a thought about something happening, then it might happen.
    a. *Example:* "I had the image that we ran over an animal when driving home, so we need to go back and check for dead animals on the road."
    b. *Example:* "If I think about hurting my brother then I probably did, and now I need to check on him to make sure he is OK."

▸ **Superstitious Thinking:** By thinking or doing something, I will cause or prevent something else from happening.

    a. *Example:* "If I wash my hands 33 times a day, then my parents will be safe."

    b. *Example:* "If I knock twice with my left hand and twice with my right hand and say a prayer, nothing bad will happen to me."

▸ **Magical Thinking:** Thinking some things are lucky and some things are unlucky, such as numbers.

    a. *Example:* "The number six is lucky, so I will buy the sixth magazine, take just the sixth tissue, pack six pairs of socks."

    b. *Example:* "There are good signs and bad signs. If I hear a certain song, that means something bad will happen, so I need to compensate by counting to 100 and backward from 100."

The OCD Workbook: Your Guide to Breaking Free From Obsessive-Compulsive Disorder (Hyman & Pedrick, 2005), written for adults, summarized the OCD cycle. The four parts of the cycle (in order) are: "(1) activating event, (2) unrealistic appraisal of the event, (3) excessive anxiety, and (4) neutralizing ritual" (Hyman & Pedrick, 2005, p. 100). Let me go through a few examples, using the numbers to identify the steps:

▸ (1) use a public restroom, (2) obsessive thought that restrooms have many bad germs and that these bad germs will get on me and I will get sick or will get cancer, (3) very anxious, and (4) wash hands thoroughly with lots of soap.

▸ (1) walk by an abandoned bag on the street, (2) irrational thought that the bag has toxic airborne substance in it, (3) very anxious, and (4) ask Mom over and over for reassurance that I did not get sick from passing the bag on the street.

▶ (1) walking on sidewalk, (2) obsessive thought that I stepped on a bug and killed it and God will see me as a bad person, (3) very anxious, and (4) go back and check sidewalk and sides of sidewalk multiple times; be "really good" for rest of the day to make up for sin of killing bug; pray for an hour that night.

▶ (1) going up the stairs at home, (2) thought that it doesn't "feel right" to walk up this way, (3) anxious/uncomfortable/unsettled feeling, and (4) go back and walk up in a different way, then go back and walk up in another way, multiple times until it "feels right," and then go upstairs.

▶ (1) Mom says goodnight at bedtime, (2) she didn't say "I love you" in the right way—it felt rushed and not real, (3) anxious, and (4) have Mom repeat goodnight and say "I love you" several times until she says it "right."

Understanding the OCD cycle helps your child externalize the OCD and can give him greater awareness of his experience with OCD. I recommend teaching your child about the cycle and going through a few examples with him.

Children can have limited or no insight into the irrationality of their obsessive thoughts and still be diagnosed with OCD (whereas adults do need to recognize it). It often is the case where a child lacks insight into his or her OCD and does not question the meaning or relevance of it, but they just do the rituals. OCD also can appear as very odd behavior, such as hoarding trash or food under one's bed, touching one's ear in a repetitive way, or walking in and out of a room over and over. Regardless of how strange the behaviors can appear, it's just OCD and is just as treatable as less unusual behaviors such as excessive hand washing.

When helping your child overcome OCD, it is most important for him to do loop recordings and uncertainty training recordings. This, along with behavioral exposure to anxiety-provoking/OCD situations *without* doing the typical ritual response (all listed on the ladder), is what is curative for OCD. The exposure without doing the rituals or compulsions is called Exposure/Response Prevention (E/RP), as the child is exposed to the situation he fears or has an obsession about (e.g., touching a doorknob) without doing his typical response (e.g., washing his hands, using hand sanitizer, using his sleeve, or wiping his hands on his clothes). With practice, just as the child with separation anxiety becomes comfortable sleeping in his own bed on his own, the child with OCD will become comfortable with touching doorknobs without following it with the compulsive behaviors/rituals. In addition, the research shows that the more extreme the exposures, the better the outcome. So, for the child who fears contracting germs and illness from touching doorknobs, she would touch 10 different doorknobs, then eat a sandwich without washing or doing any cleaning rituals beforehand and she would do this every day for 2 weeks, or until it no longer triggered any anxiety. Ultimately, she *habituates* to the anxiety-provoking situations just like in other anxiety disorders; the additional component is ensuring that she does it without doing her rituals/compulsions. As stated in Chapter 4, when making worry loop tapes, children with the "need to confess" compulsion will need to be limited to how many times they add recordings, as doing so can serve as the ritual (e.g., "if I confess on the tape, then I'm OK"). For these children, doing a maximum of five different loop recordings is a reasonable goal.

In Chapter 5, the detached mindfulness technique described (part of metacognitive therapy, or MCT) is another important strategy to use when your child has OCD, as it helps externalize the OCD thoughts and also helps to reclassify the thoughts as symptoms of the OCD. This is another way to help your child take the power away from her anxious thoughts (remember that thoughts don't have any power, except the power we give them). Many times, OCD causes your child to doubt who she is, and detached mindfulness helps to reframe thoughts as "just thoughts," not a real reflection that deserves consideration. Instead of examining the content of the thoughts (participating in them), children learn how to see the thoughts from observer-mode and learn that OCD thoughts have no power and are irrelevant. They learn to say, "Oh, there I go again, having an OCD thought." They learn to reclassify the thoughts as OCD symptoms.

Another metacognitive therapy technique is called Attention Training Technique (ATT). I have found this particularly beneficial for children with OCD and tend to recommend it after they have completed the worry tape practice, as it is too time consuming to do both at the same time. ATT is a 12-minute long exercise to be completed twice a day, ideally. The child listens to a script and is instructed to focus on different sounds, then to switch his attention from one sound to another, and then to count all the sounds he hears at the same time (during which all of the previous sounds occur at the same time). The script is found on the MCT Institute website (see references) and is also in Dr. Adrian Wells's book (it can be recorded by you, or your child's therapist). With repeated listening, your child is trained to easily switch from one thought (sound) to another, which addresses the common problem of being stuck, or locked into, a thought. Dr. Wells considers anxiety and OCD to be a "cognitive attentional syndrome" in which the person's attention gets stuck on an unwanted or anxiety-provoking thought (as a note, this has nothing to do with ADHD). His techniques of detached mindfulness and Attention Training Technique are designed to break this attention and enable the child to stop the rumination cycle. As with the other CBT strategies in this book, these MCT techniques are also empirically supported and proven to work.

All parents of children with anxiety unintentionally reinforce, or strengthen it, by accommodating it; however, when it comes to parents of OCD, this tendency is even greater. Research on family accommodation of children with OCD has linked the accommodation with both severity of the child's OCD and stress of the family, meaning that both are worse when there is accommodation (Storch et al., 2007). Chapter 12 provides guidance on how to replace your natural tendency to accommodate and temporarily relieve your child's distress with a more effective and supportive approach, including what to say to your child when he comes to you for reassurance.

Compared to anxiety disorders, OCD tends to have more of a genetic component (runs in family). For this reason, of the conditions I treat, OCD tends to be more likely to require medication (typically SSRIs), and this is usually prescribed to reduce the thoughts that come up with OCD. However, it is important to keep in mind that much research shows that children and adults with OCD who are treated only with medication and not CBT or other therapy do not do nearly as well as those who have CBT treatment, whether that treatment occurs alone without medication or in addition to medication (Association for Behavioral and Cognitive Therapies, n.d.). The positive outcomes from CBT are longer lasting (even after therapy has been discontinued), whereas medication must be continued to achieve the benefit. Although the study led by John Walkup (Walkup et al., 2008; cited in Chapter 1) found 55% of the children improved on medication alone during the 14-week treatment period, we cannot know how long lasting these results are; the study also supported a combination of CBT and medication over medication alone.

Panic Disorder (PD)

The first step in helping a child who suffers from panic attacks is teaching her to label the panic attack itself. Labeling it helps your child know the symptoms of panic and normalize what is happening. Initially, you will label the panic attack for her and then reassure your child that she can handle it and that the very unpleasant panic sensations will pass (no one in the history of the world has ever stayed stuck in a panic attack!).

The key to overcoming panic is to learn how to "ride the wave" of panic (and as her parent, you will coach her on how to do this). This in and of itself actually will lessen the severity of the panic. She needs to learn to be able to tolerate and not fear the symptoms. Panic is a frightening experience and it becomes worsened by the worry that one is panicking: The child with panic is most anxious about the fact that he is panicking—it truly is a "fear of fear." Yet, the panic attack itself is not threatening or damaging (just very uncomfortable and unpleasant). Knowing what is happening and knowing how to cope with it makes the attack less severe. Plus, accepting that it is happening typically will cause it to pass in a shorter time.

The opposite of accepting the panic attack and "riding the wave" is trying to get out of it. This actually worsens the panic and empowers the panic's power over your child. For this reason, using calm breathing during a panic attack is contraindicated: If you try to calm down during a panic attack, it doesn't work and ends up making the panic more frightening because you can't get out of it. The child reacts to being unable to breathe calmly, and typically ends up hyperventilating even more, mentally reflecting "what's wrong with me . . . why can't I calm my breathing?" The better method is to stop the anxious reaction to the panic attack itself; essentially, eliminating the fear of the fear. When she learns how to tolerate the discomfort, the fear will start to feel manageable and the attacks will be less severe and shorter in duration.

When children continually worry about having panic attacks, then it resembles more of a panic disorder and causes avoidance behavior (e.g., they start missing events due to a fear of having a panic attack in that situation). For these children, they benefit from uncertainty training ("It's always possible that I'll have a panic attack. It's always possible that it will go on for a long time and I won't be able to get out of it.") in addition to the exposure work.

Behavioral exposure to panic is very effective; this is when your child deliberately induces the panic symptoms (the ultimate example of an anxiety-provoking situation) in a systematic way. It teaches them that they don't have to be afraid of the panic. To practice the symptoms, I start by having children deliberately "hyperventilate" (breathe in and out rapidly and loudly for 30–45 seconds) and allow them to tolerate the discomfort. Once we complete this exercise and they have been able to handle the uncomfortable feelings, I will have them practice hyperventilating, then do calm breathing right after, just for the purposes of showing them the range of how we breathe and how each form of breathing makes them feel: On one end of the continuum is hyperventilation and on the other end is natural, calm breathing (I remind them, however, that they still should not use calm breathing during an actual panic attack). Other ways of inducing symptoms include running and up and down the stairs (rapid heartbeat) and then turning around in circles (dizziness), and breathing in and out through a very small straw (difficulty breathing). Practicing the symptoms can be included on their ladder, as this is how they are facing their fears: "Practice anxious breathing," "Practice feeling dizzy," "Practice having a fast heartbeat." Then, if there is avoidance of certain situations or places due to a fear of having a panic attack, these situations should be listed as steps on the ladder. A great reference on this approach is *Facing Panic* by R. Reid Wilson (2003; available at http://www.adaa.org). Originally written for adults, I successfully apply the concepts of this book to my work with children.

Like OCD, panic attacks occur in a cycle. R. Reid Wilson (2003) does a fantastic job of explaining the cycle, which has four parts: "(1) anticipatory anxiety, (2) panic attack, (3) escape and relief, and (4) self-doubt and self-criticism" (p. 6). Not all children with panic necessarily go though these four stages, but the cycle describes what many experience. The anticipatory anxiety (e.g., "Oh, no! What if I have a panic attack at school?") increases a child's anxiety level and he worries about an impending panic attack, which increases the likelihood of a panic attack. Once the panic attack occurs, the idea of leaving the situation is linked with feeling a strong sense of relief ("I have to go home"). Following this escape/relief, an experience of self-doubt and feeling badly about oneself comes up. For example, I worked with a child who would get very anxious about going to school. He would work himself up into a panic attack (it always started with anticipatory anxiety the night before a school day, but was particularly worse in the morning and once he arrived at school). By first period, he would be in a full-blown panic attack and would go to the school nurse who promptly called his mother (at his request) to pick him up. His mother, a caring woman who had genuine concern for her child's health, quickly came to school and inadvertently reinforced (and worsened) his anxiety. Once he was home, he would feel embarrassed and "like a failure" because he couldn't stay in school "like everyone else." During his treatment with me, he learned that he needed to stay in school no matter what—even if he needed to take a break from classes to go to the nurse's office—he needed to return to class once he felt a bit calmer.

Once your child has completed this program, if any future panic arises, you should help her label the panic attack and encourage her to reassure herself (e.g., asking "What do you think is going on for you right now?" cues her that it is panic) and use her coping strategies. Finally, it is noteworthy that many children with panic attacks are sensitive to minor changes in their bodies, such as shortness of breath or increased heartbeat (and often mislabel these as symptoms of panic), thus it will be helpful for you to explain that there are normal fluctuations in the body and that these changes are not of concern.

In sum, the most important goals in overcoming panic are (1) not panicking about panicking, (2) tolerating the unpleasant feelings and physical sensations, and (3) not avoiding activities or situations because of a fear of panic or a panic attack itself.

Tips on Other Anxiety-Driven Behaviors or Problems

Perfectionism

Perfectionism often is a developmentally appropriate character-istic in childhood: Children are socialized to understand that there is a right way and a wrong way to do things, that things should be done in a certain order, that they should clean up after themselves, and so on. This type of learning is appropriate and necessary. Therefore, children can show perfectionistic traits when attempting to "follow the rules." However, there comes a time when flexibility and the ability to consider alternatives to the usual way of doing things becomes important, and essential. For perfectionistic chil-dren, they don't acquire this flexibility, or it may be limited; they often display rigidity and inflexibility that then results in frustra-tion and disappointment. Perfectionism can be focused on grades, how they dress, or how their things are arranged.

Perfectionistic children tend to have excessively high and unre-alistic expectations for themselves (and sometimes for others), be inflexible and rigid, frequently make social comparisons, and have difficulty delegating tasks to others because they want to ensure it is done their way ("correctly"). They often seek reassurance and validation from others, have trouble making decisions, overcheck their work, may avoid risks due to a fear of failure, and spend exces-sive time organizing and list-making.

Perfectionistic children often have to have things a certain way in order to feel OK, and typically have a hard time accepting that there is more than one way to do something. For example, they tend to be overly concerned with the right and wrong and insist that things be done in the "right" way. A child who spends 3 hours on a writing assignment that should take no more than 45 minutes because he needs every line to be scholarly and every word precise is demonstrating extreme perfectionism. Another example is the child who won't let anyone go into her room in fear that they might move something around and she won't know what was touched or moved. Helping children learn to replace these thoughts and behaviors with healthier, more balanced ones is part of the process of change. These rigid and inflexible approaches to dealing with life events should be challenged in the same spirit as the other anxiety behaviors are challenged. Thus, they should be integrated into the child's ladder and practiced in the same way. For instance, a step on the ladder could be "get a B on a quiz on purpose," "miss the bus one day," "have your brother go in your room and move something to a different place," or "keep something in your room 'out of place' for a day." These examples give perfectionistic children the experience of learning that things are still OK if they are done differently, even if its not done in the "right" or "best" or "usual" way. The practices also help to, as my good colleague Dr. Charlie Manseuto says, "Welcome the child to the world of the 'good enough.'" For example, children who must have everything excessively organized in their room at all times at the expense of having playtime learn that they could skip putting every single thing away in its place and leave a part of the room temporarily cluttered and play with their neighbor instead of cleaning. When it comes to keeping their room a certain way, they learn that they can be "good enough" about it with no repercussions. Sometimes we turn in an assignment that is "good enough" instead of asking for an extension.

Challenging the child's perfectionistic thoughts also is important. All-or-nothing thinking and "shoulds" tend to organize the child's cognitive life in addition to how he behaves. In the Resources section, I have included a book called *When Perfect Isn't Good Enough* by Martin Antony and Richard Swinson. This book provides excellent descriptions of the common perfectionistic thoughts and behaviors and although it is written for adults (and older teens), it certainly applies to the understanding of perfectionism in children, and parents will benefit from reviewing it (although it would need to be verbally adapted for children to understand).

Being Easily Overwhelmed

Many anxious children get overwhelmed easily, and this tendency to be overwhelmed often centers on school—classwork, homework, and tests. When this happens, the overwhelmed feeling actually makes the task longer and seem worse and more intensive; this can cause the child to procrastinate. If your child experiences this, try helping her develop the daily behavior of creating "To do" checklists, in which she lists out the subjects and the homework in each. Help her to be "in the moment," and only focus on the task at hand. For example, you can make her a self-talk note card that reads: "I need to be in the present moment and only focus on one thing at a time," "When I only focus on the assignment I am working on, I am OK, " or "The only thing that will make me feel better is doing the work, so let me get to it and focus my energy only on doing the task itself, not on thinking about it." Uncertainty training (described above under the GAD section) also can be used for this issue to help the overwhelming thoughts be less of a trigger; for example, your child can practice repeating: "It is always possible that I won't finish all of my work." With repetition, scary thoughts will be neutralized and will no longer create that alarming anxious feeling.

You might need to monitor her approach to doing her homework and help her organize the assignments, perhaps breaking down assignments into smaller steps so they seem more manageable. When you see your child becoming overwhelmed, encourage her to take a 10-minute break to calm down, reminding her that in a calm state, she is more efficient, and then return to doing her work with a more relaxed attitude. If this can be done repetitively, your child will soon begin to associate doing homework with being calm. Otherwise, if your child continues to focus on her work while her heart is beating and she is rushing and nervous, she will associate homework with being anxious.

Many children experience test anxiety. This can cause a huge interference for your child, and may even cause your child to blank out and score poorly on exams. Relaxation techniques, uncertainty training, challenging catastrophic thinking, and creating steps on the ladder to expose your child to test situations will help your child overcome his test anxiety. The ladder exposures can include practice tests at home, practice timed tests at home, and working collaboratively with teachers to let your child take a pretest (a test before the real test on similar content area). For text anxiety, I find the exposure practices plus pairing one-nostril breathing with tests to be most effective.

Finally, it can be helpful to use a calendar and stickers to note each day that your child approaches his homework in a calm and collected way. This provides a way to track his progress and also redefines success as being calm and relaxed and puts the focus on the approach taken toward doing homework, rather than the focus on finishing all of the work perfectly.

Excessive Guilt

Some children, most of who have generalized anxiety or OCD exhibit the symptom of excessive guilt. Although the emotion of guilt can be useful in that it can represent one's conscience and keep the person "in check" with his or her values, *excessive* guilt serves no purpose, other than to make the person feel miserable. Children who have excessive guilt may repeatedly say, "I feel bad about" or "I feel bad when I," and get triggered into feeling guilty (and often anxious) from meaningless events. For example, Melissa, a bright and very kind 13-year-old, felt bad every time her parents bought her something. She needed new cleats for soccer and when simply reminding her mother that she needed them, she was triggered into intense feelings of guilt. Sometimes she would feel so bad that she would cry. As a typical teenager, Melissa enjoyed getting new things and appreciated dressing nicely; however, this enjoyment was compromised by her contrasting feelings of excessive guilt, fueled by thoughts of disadvantaged children who have less. What should have been a pleasurable experience became a source of much distress and unhappiness. In this way, Melissa's guilt caused an interference in her life. In the course of her treatment with me, Melissa shared tons of things that made her feel guilty, such as forgetting to say goodnight to her babysitter, being annoyed with one of her classmates (a normal experience for most kids), going shopping with her parents, and getting a reward from her mother for reading a book.

Melissa and I identified her thinking errors, which included "shoulds" ("I should never forget to say goodnight to the babysitter," "I should not have nice things when there are all these poor people in the world"), all-or-nothing thinking ("If I get new clothes, then I'm not being sensitive to disadvantaged children," and selective attention ("I'm not as considerate as I could be . . . I didn't even say goodnight to the sitter"), and then made a worry loop recording (over several sessions—doing it on different days was very helpful) of *everything* she felt guilty or bad about. I instructed her to listen to the tape over and over for at least 15 minutes each day. Within a month of doing this, Melissa's guilty thoughts went away, and they stayed away! Several months later, she even commented with both surprise and excitement, "I don't feel bad anymore!" The excitement in her voice reflected her newfound freedom. When children feel bad and anxious, they are robbed of the freedom to simply enjoy life. Gaining freedom from this, and a stronger sense of confidence about herself and her feelings (because she no longer doubted or questioned herself, which the guilt caused her to do), was liberating for Melissa.

If your child experiences excessive guilt, you also can make a recording with him of all of the things that he feels guilty about and then play the recording repeatedly like Melissa did. The main goal of the tape is twofold: (1) to help your child externalize his emotions, taking the emotion from inside his mind to outside of himself and (2) to help him *habituate*, or become used to his guilt-provoking or distressing thoughts. Finally, it is beneficial to make your child some self-talk note cards on this subject. Some examples include: "Feeling guilty when I did not do anything wrong is useless," and "Everyone makes mistakes. No one is perfect, including me." I love this quote from *Stick Up for Yourself!: Every Kid's Guide to Personal Power and Positive Self-Esteem:* "Feelings aren't right or wrong, good or bad. Feelings just are" (Kaufman, Raphael, & Espeland, 1999, pg. 24).

Health Anxiety

Children with health anxiety include those who are hyperfocused on physical symptoms, preoccupied with the notion that something health-wise is wrong, and often complain of something wrong with their health. They may seek or try to seek medical help or treatment, and even hope to find that something is wrong in order to explain their symptoms. Although health anxiety most often is a part of either GAD or OCD, it can be a problem in and of itself. Initially, I often refer these children for a physical exam to rule out true medical problems (although many have already undergone comprehensive testing by the time I work with them). I recommend the medical exam for two reasons: (1) children with health anxiety still get sick and can have medical issues just as children without health anxiety do, and (2) this allows me to refer to fact-based evidence that they are healthy and treat it as anxiety, so that I can address the "symptoms" as anxiety symptoms.

The best recommendation I can make to parents is to strike a balance between showing compassion and not enabling or validating the child (e.g., allowing the child to miss school or other obligations) or accommodating the fears or reinforcing the health anxiety (e.g., providing reassurance that the symptom is not an issue, repeatedly bringing him to the doctor, letting him sleep in your bed when he is complaining of not feeling well). Whether or not there is a real problem and whether or not your child consciously is using physical complaints in a manipulative way, your child is still struggling with feeling OK. The balance is responding to this struggle and her worries in a caring and loving way without reinforcing her beliefs and behaviors. Try to establish a pattern of the worry to help identify if there is something stressing her.

Finally, I have children with health anxiety complete a Daily Log of Health Concerns (there is a good one in the book by Taylor and Asmundson, see the Resources section), which requires them to record if they worried that day about a health-related symptom or illness, how strong/intense the worry was, if they avoided anything due to worry or concern, and any other behavior such as reassurance-seeking or looking up symptoms that they may have done. Over a period of 3–4 weeks, the child usually ends up having about 20 or so logs, many of which demonstrate that the worry is constant and that no bad outcomes came from the worry (in other words, that "bump" on their arm went away, they didn't have internal bleeding, etc.). The Daily Log offers good evidence that the issue is one of anxiety, not of physical disease. Once they have 20 or so of these logs completed, I will have them put it in a binder that they can reference when future concerns come up. Usually, they will see a log form has already been completed for that same feared symptom (e.g., there might be 10 forms already filled out for "found a bump"), which gives them validation that their worries are due to health anxiety rather than a true medical issue.

Hair Pulling

Hair pulling, called *trichotillomania* or trich for short, is a repetitive behavior disorder in which the individual pulls hair from her head or scalp, eyebrows, eyelashes, or other parts of her body. This is distinguished from other "picking" habits such as nail biting or picking skin, as it is exclusive to hair and typically more complex. The hair pulling behavior can feel like an addiction and there is a tactile (touch) sensation to the pulling of the hair that is strongly reinforced each time the child pulls. Bald spots or missing eyebrows or lashes are common and this can cause the person to feel socially embarrassed. Hair pulling is best treated with professional help. As it is beyond the scope of this book, I have provided recommended books in the Resources section for this topic.

School Refusal Behavior

School refusal behavior can be a symptom of severe social anxiety and tends to cause a significant interference that can go on for years and create tremendous distress for the child and the whole family. Alternatively, school refusal can be a form of oppositional defiant disorder (ODD; see the Resources section under Parenting and Discipline). Although this topic is not a focal point of the book, I will make a few suggestions based on my work with this population of children. Frankly, this is one of the most challenging problems to address, but I have worked with many successful cases, so I encourage you to stay hopeful about a solution to this problem.

First and foremost, the child's school and parents need to work collaboratively on addressing this problem. There needs to be a contact person at the child's school who is willing to check in daily with the parents and who the child will report to when she attends school or when she does not (e.g., call from home). When there is a therapist involved in the treatment process, that therapist should work closely with the school as well. If possible, a multidisciplinary team meeting with the parents, therapist, school counselor/teachers/principal, and possibly the child (depending on the age—children 10 and above should attend and younger children can, as well, although there should be some discussion about it), should be arranged at the school.

Second, parents will need to alter their parenting approach, particularly when it comes to discipline. School refusal behavior typically includes an oppositional component and many children with this issue also meet the criteria for an oppositional defiant disorder. Many parents of kids with ODD end up permitting behavior they normally would find unacceptable. Researchers have identified four types of parenting styles, all described by the amount of warmth and the amount of demand/expectations that parents place upon their children (Baumrind, 1971, 1991; Maccoby & Martin, 1983). The four types and descriptions are as follows, going from most demand placed on the child to least demand placed on the child but not in order of rank: authoritarian (high demand, low warmth), authoritative (high demand, high warmth), permissive (low demand, high warmth), and uninvolved (low demand, low warmth). The type that has been found to be the best is the authoritative type (high demand, high warmth); these are parents who are empathic and sensitive to their child's emotions and offer warmth and concern, yet they have expectations for their child and will provide appropriate and reasonable discipline and consequences when these expectations are not met. The type that I find occurs most often in families with children who refuse to attend school is the permissive type. When working with these families, I typically do separate sessions with the parent(s) and help them develop an attitude of expectations and authority while maintaining empathy and warmth. Too many children in these families believe that it is their *choice* to attend or not to attend school. Scott Sells, author of *Parenting Your Out-of-Control Teenager: 7 Steps to Reestablish Authority and Reclaim Love* (2002), identified that one of the biggest problems is unclear rules. Many families with school refusal children do not communicate the rule that children must attend school, and that attending school is nonnegotiable. The message parents need to give is that attending school is not an option—it is a rule! Just as adults have to go to work, children need to go to school—it is their job. And, just as adults who choose not to go to work suffer the consequences (e.g., no money, no new clothes, no entertainment), children who choose not to go to school also should have these consequences (of course, removal of food and/

or shelter should never be included in these consequences). When kids end up getting to stay home in their pajamas watching TV or playing on their computer, it reinforces the school avoidance. The alternative to not going to school needs to be less pleasant (going to the library all day, volunteering at a shelter all day, etc.). I've had parents disconnect the Internet and remove TV cables with great outcomes; I've had successful parents say to their child, "Home is closed during school hours!"

Third, learning disabilities (LD) or learning differences need to be considered as contributing factors in a child's refusal to go to school. Some children with school refusal have underlying dyslexia or auditory processing problems that make it hard for them to understand what they are learning and to do the work in the time allotted. It might be necessary to have your child tested for learning differences. If he has an LD, the school is required to create an IEP (Individualized Education Program) for your child, giving him the accommodations he needs to attain academic success.

Fourth, what initially caused the school refusal behavior and what maintains it may not be the same. Once a significant amount of school has been missed, the child loses his sense of belonging in the school and typically feels lost in the classroom and isolated socially. I recommend that you give your child assurance that once he returns to school on a daily (thus, consistent) basis, these issues will dissolve. He will catch up academically (ideally, the school will make some accommodations and reduce the amount of make-up work) and he will improve socially. The most important idea for your child to grasp is that there is only one solution: to go to school! This problem will not be resolved and will not go away until he goes to school on time every day. Stress inoculation really helps prepare children in their return to school and includes going through a sample dialogue back and forth regarding what other kids may ask or say, what they can say in response, what the other kids will then ask or say, what they will then say, and so on, until you have rehearsed four sets of back-and-forth communication. Most of the time, kids will ask where the child has been (the child can reply, "I've been sick, but I'm better now") and then they move on without more questions. Stress inoculation training is most helpful in reducing the child's anticipatory anxiety about returning to school.

Selective Mutism

As stated above, selective mutism is not addressed in-depth in this book (see the Resources section for recommended books on this topic). Selective mutism is a less common form of social phobia in which the child refuses to speak in certain circumstances (e.g., in particular situations or when around specific people) but speaks freely and openly, often in an extroverted way, in other circumstances. For example, a child with selective mutism may remain completely silent at school and avoid all eye contact but once at home, she will brighten up and speak freely in a loud voice, often openly stating opinions and preferences. One misconception about children with selective mutism is that, because they are not talking, they are not communicating. On the contrary, these children communicate quite a bit nonverbally. One child I worked with who had selective mutism did not speak to me at all for eight sessions, yet, starting at the fourth meeting, she brought in artwork and dolls to show me and her eye contact gradually increased. Although these children can be painfully slow to warm up to new people and become comfortable in new situations, research supports a CBT approach with systematic desensitization (using the step-by-step ladder exposures as a guide).

Bedwetting

Bedwetting sometimes can be a manifestation of anxiety, although it often is not caused by anxiety. If your child is wetting, it is important to consult with your pediatrician and rule out any physical problems before psychological causes are considered. Regardless of the causes, under no circumstances should children be shamed or criticized for wetting the bed. However, children can be involved in either cleaning up after the wetting or assisting in the clean-up, as this can (but does not always) reduce his embarrassment because he took part in remedying the situation. Please refer to a book on this subject listed in the Resources section for more information.

Tips on Handling Your Child's Anxiety With Others

Another issue that comes up for parents of children with anxiety is how to handle informing others of the anxiety problem. This includes what to say to other parents and children; managing play dates, parties, and sleepovers; and working with other parents when their own child becomes part of the exposure practice (e.g., if one of your child's steps on the ladder is to have a sleepover).

Other parents generally will be understanding when you explain that your child has an anxiety problem; remember that all children experience anxiety at some point in their lives. The more factual you are, the better. Explain that your child has anxiety about _____ (separation, social events, sleepovers, dogs), and that you and your child are working on this problem. Explain that you are arranging "practices" for him to learn how to face his fears, and that you would really appreciate their support.

For example, let's say that your child has either separation anxiety or social anxiety and is invited to a sleepover party. Talking with the parent who is throwing the party is necessary. Once you explain about the anxiety, tell the other parent that your child has strategies that he can use, such as calm breathing and positive self-talk, and that while he may be anxious at first, he will become comfortable soon. If the other parent is comfortable (and you trust that he or she can handle it), he or she can tell your child, "I spoke with your mom (or dad) and I know that you are working on feeling better about sleepovers. If you are having a hard time, please let me know." This gives your child the sense that there is someone else who is temporarily on her team and who can offer support if needed. The other parent should know that if your child does approach him or her, any discussion of your child's anxiety should occur in private. You can make a plan with your child and the other parent that if it becomes too hard for your child, he can give a cue to the other parent and together they can call you for additional support. Your child should know that while he is strongly discouraged from leaving the sleepover (as this can strengthen the avoidance behavior), in a worst-case scenario, you will come and pick him up. The reason for this is that, unless totally necessary, no child should be *forced* to do any of the exposures, as this can make her even more anxious to face her fears and reinforce a sense of disempowerment or helplessness. During the exposure practice, she needs to know that she has a way out of a scary situation if it becomes too much for her to handle. Usually, most ladders should include several gradual steps for sleepovers, such as going to the party but leaving just before bedtime. Again, while I do not condone fibbing or lying, I think it is perfectly reasonable that your child have the option of keeping the fact that he is facing his fears a private matter. Thus, making up excuses while doing the ladder should be an option. For instance, in the case where your child leaves before bedtime, he can tell the other children that he has a family event the next day that requires him to get up really early to attend, and so he needs to sleep at home. Also, if he needs to leave early, he can make the excuse that he is not feeling well. This helps to prevent feeling further isolated from peers and additionally stressed about what to say. As a general rule, the more you plan out the exposure, including preparing your child for what he could say in a variety of different scenarios (like the stress inoculation), the better off you (and he!) will be.

Sometimes your child will show signs of anxiety while in the presence of other children, for example, when on a play date.

The same recommendation to be factual applies and you can say, "Sally has a phobia of dogs, which means she is afraid of them, but she is working to get rid of it. I know it might be hard to understand since you love dogs, but some kids are very afraid of them." With anxiety disorders other than phobias, it is best to *describe* the symptom rather than using the terms "obsessive-compulsive disorder" or "separation anxiety disorder." For instance, you can say, "Sometimes Ruth gets nervous about sharing food with other people, but she is working on it," or "Sometimes Thelma has a hard time doing things alone, but she is working on it." This helps to describe the behavior and identify it as a problem that is being addressed. I recommend that this approach be used with friends of your child and not simply acquaintances or children that may tease others. Most children will appreciate the clarification and not question it.

One Last Thought for Parents

First, I want to congratulate you again for taking this important and proactive step of helping your child with his anxiety. As a parent, it is extremely painful to watch your child experience fear and discomfort, which is generally part of the picture with an anxious child. Many parents worry about being responsible for their child's anxiety disorder, and feel conflicted about how to handle it—swaying between an instinct to comfort and soothe their child and a desire to challenge him and make him stronger. The purpose of this book has been to give you guidance on how to best manage this fine line and how to help your child overcome his fears. Even if you end up needing professional support to treat your child's anxiety, starting with this book is something to be proud of. I also want to reassure you that, while anxiety can have genetic influences, many do not; either way, parents do not cause anxious disorders. Although modeling anxious responses has been found to be a possible contributor to the development of anxiety, most of the time it simply "just shows up" as its own problem.

Overcoming anxiety, as delineated in this program, can foster resilience in children, as they learn how to problem solve, face difficult situations, and take a proactive approach. On a personal note, dealing with and working through my own childhood experience of loss and the resulting separation anxiety helped prepare me for the future and made me a stronger and more resilient person. Obviously, it also made me a believer in therapy and self-help! Not only do children benefit from overcoming their fears, but they often are more therapy-friendly as they have either completed this program as a "self-help" approach led by me, a psychologist, or in the context of a therapeutic relationship with a mental health professional. Being familiar with therapy in childhood can make it easier to use it as a resource or reference in adulthood.

CHAPTER

11

Anxiety at Bedtime

Improving Sleep Behavior

I FREQUENTLY give talks to local schools on how parents can help children cope with anxiety and stress; never have I given a talk where I wasn't asked at least one question about sleep and the anxiety that comes up at bedtime for so many children. Difficulty falling asleep, staying asleep, and sleeping in their own bed are common issues in childhood. In fact, having trouble with sleep during childhood is the rule, rather than the exception. Much of the time, the child may have separation anxiety or fears about bad things happening at night. Just like other anxiety, the goal is to help your child face her bedtime fears.

Before I explain my approach to getting children to fall asleep comfortably and confidently on their own in their bed and staying in it throughout the night, it is important to clarify that this chapter applies to families who: (1) would like their children to sleep separately, and (2) their children have anxiety about doing so. The research on family co-sleeping (bed shared by parent[s] and child) shows that it does *not* have any negative impact on the child; short- and long-term, these children thrive just as well and are just as confident and attached as those who sleep on their own (see http://www.askdrsears.com for more information). There could be an impact on the marital unit, of course, as having children in your bed can pose an obstacle to alone time with one's partner. This chapter addresses the problem that occurs when you want your child to fall asleep without you (in their bed, not yours), but you struggle to get this to happen due to their anxiety and fears. This struggle can cause a great deal of stress and impair your well-being.

Treating bedtime fears is often a challenge for parents due to several factors (e.g., guilt, tendency to accommodate, exhaustion). It requires a great deal of emotional strength and perseverance on part of the parent. Many just succumb to the anxiety and resign to letting their children sleep with them, even though they wish for a different arrangement. It helps to focus on two motivating factors: (1) quality sleep is imperative for physical and mental health, and (2) children become more confident when they overcome anxiety and its barriers.

The importance of sleep cannot be underestimated. Sleep deprivation has been linked with memory issues, symptoms of inattention, weakened immune system and less ability to fight off colds, poor glucose absorption (e.g., putting individuals at risk for diabetes and weight gain), and a greater likelihood of experiencing stress and negative mood states. People without ADHD who are sleep deprived (6 hours or less) show similar PET scan (brain scan while doing a task) results to those of individuals with ADHD; they show the same underactivation in the prefrontal cortex section of the brain, which is associated with working memory, attention, organization, and other abilities (Goel, Rao, Durmer, & Dinges, 2009). Given all of these robust findings associated with sleep, parents need to be highly motivated and disciplined about getting their child to form healthy sleep habits and behaviors, and not allow anxiety to cause an interference in what is an essential component of health. When there is anxiety at bedtime, including fears of being alone, fears of break-ins, fears of being kidnapped, and separation anxiety from parents, it creates a behavioral problem for children and their parents.

Common anxious behaviors at bedtime include:

- ▶ wanting a parent present when falling asleep;

- ▶ refusing to sleep alone in their bed;
- ▶ repeatedly leaving their room to get a parent;
- ▶ coming to the parent's bed in the middle of the night;
- ▶ seeking reassurance that nothing bad will happen;
- ▶ insisting on specific "good night" rituals, including how the parent says good night;
- ▶ checking the locks, doors, and windows, checking on pets;
- ▶ sleeping in a certain position (e.g., facing the door); and
- ▶ needing doors to remain open or closed or lights to be on.

The approach is similar to sleep training, in which the parent gradually removes him- or herself from helping the child fall asleep on her own; several studies have shown sleep training to have no negative outcomes for children (Price, Wake, Ukomunne, & Hiscock, 2012). The approach is similar to general treatment of anxiety disorders, in which they no longer engage in avoidance behavior (avoidance of sleeping alone) and parents stop making accommodations (e.g., no longer reassuring their child that it will be OK, that no one will break in and kidnap them, etc.). Just like other children with anxiety who face their fears, children who conquer their fears around bedtime develop a strong self-confidence resulting from overcoming their anxiety. The parental role in tackling this behavior is essential, and the need for consistent responding is paramount.

Start by explaining to your child that it is time to conquer the sleep issue; you can give some information on the importance of sleep and how the anxiety about bedtime is making everyone lose sleep, but the emphasis is really on this being an anxious behavior to overcome (facing her fears). Set a date for the plan to start; many families have found it helpful to start on a Friday or other day followed by a few days of no school. Several children have started after there has been some time away from home, either on vacation or going on an overnight trip with school. It can also be helpful for siblings to sleep out for 2–3 nights, if possible, so your devotion to the plan is not compromised by concern about waking your other child(ren). Prepare for the plan by getting a calendar that will be used to track her progress, as you will award stars for each night she sleeps on her own (not in your bed, not with you; give a star even if she falls asleep on the floor outside your door). Review the general strategies she can use if she is anxious or has trouble falling asleep (relaxation strategies, mindfulness techniques, self-talk) and make a handout for your child called "What To Do When You Cannot Fall Asleep" like the one below.

What To Do When You Cannot Fall Asleep

1. Try relaxation: Do calm breathing, progressive muscle relaxation, or use relaxing imagery.
2. Read self-talk cards.
3. Use distraction: Make lists using the ABCs (boy's names: Adam, Brian, Cole, Dan, Ed; jobs: artist, baker, chef, dentist, engineer; fruit/veggies: apple, banana, carrot, date, eggplant; or cities/states/countries: Africa, Baltimore, Chicago, Delaware, Ecuador). If you get stuck on a letter, just move on.
4. Do yoga (do 2 minutes of five Yoga Pretzel cards).
5. Listen to relaxation CD or app.

Your child can also make self-talk cards for targeting sleep (add these to the standard self-talk cards from Chapter 4):

- What would someone without sleep anxiety think? What would they do? How would they feel about bedtime?
- Sleep is soothing and cozy, and my body needs to rest.
- Think about how animals sleep and how babies sleep—it's so natural for them.
- I can learn how to "just be" and relax in my body.
- I can quiet my mind and let my thoughts go. I can just be in my body and let relaxation and sleep happen.

- ▶ I cannot allow anxiety to control my life. I cannot allow anxiety to prevent me from sleeping on my own.
- ▶ If other kids can do it, so can I.
- ▶ This is my house, my room, my bed, and I won't let anxiety prevent me from feeling comfortable here. Peace is in me and I can feel peace here.

Many children have benefitted from listening to different recordings targeting relaxation at bedtime. You can install one of the apps I recommend (listed in the Resources section) on a smartphone or tablet, and then set your phone to be locked on that app (so other parts of the phone or tablet will not be used). For example, if you have an iPhone, you can initiate "Guided Access" (under Settings and General and Accessibility) and then open the app, triple click to turn it on, and then the device becomes just the app (you will need to set/use a passcode to unlock it from the Guided Access, so make it a passcode that your child cannot guess).

After fueling your child with strategies, making the "What To Do When You Cannot Fall Asleep" handout and self-talk cards for sleep, and possibly cueing up relaxation recordings, you initiate the plan:

1. Tuck your child in (relaxing routine of story, cuddle, song: 10–20 minutes max).
2. Leave the room and go into your bedroom.
3. For the first attempt to come into your room, you can walk her back to her bed (no cuddling or getting in bed with her—simply walk her back and pull the covers up with a quick kiss at most), then return to your room.
4. For the second attempt to come into your room, you stay in your doorway and wait for her to return to her room until she calls out to you once she's back in her bed. Many kids will resist this and will try to negotiate with you to have you accompany them back. Stick to the plan and do not walk her back. You can say, "I'm not walking you back.

You have a choice—I can either go back in my room now and lock the door, or I can wait here for you to walk back in and call out to me that you are back in bed." This usually causes them to walk back on their own; after they call out to you, you can say: "Great job! I love you, good night." Now you go back in your room and lock the door. (By the way, parents are never thrilled with this option, but I assure you that it is necessary and has lead to success in *every* case I've worked with on this issue.)

5. For the third attempt to come in your room (she'll knock on your locked door), you can call out from behind your door: "I love you. You can do it. Go back to your room now. Practice being brave. Read your self-talk cards. I'm going to bed now." You can say this and 1–2 additional statements, such as:

    a. "This is supposed to be hard. It's hard for every kid who learns how to be OK sleeping on their own. I understand how hard it is, but you can do it."

    b. "I know you can do this. I promise you will be so relieved in the morning."

    c. "We can't let anxiety make decisions for us. I am helping you face your fears. You can do it."

    d. "I'm proud of you. Read your handout. I love you and I'm going to bed now."

6. For the fourth or more attempts, there is no response from you. This is when parents really struggle and need to be strong. Kids can say pretty terrible things during this time, in addition to crying and screaming and pounding on your door. I've had kids say terrible things such as "I hate you. You don't love me. I wish I'd die," etc. And while all threats of hurting oneself should be taken seriously, threats that occur exclusively during sleep exposures are generally an attempt to get you to engage (real suicidal ideation doesn't

just come out during these moments of not being allowed in your room).

The worst nights are usually the first 2–3 nights, and sometimes it lasts 4–5 nights. For the majority of children, by night 5 they go to bed easily without a problem (this is when you should celebrate your great parenting!). The way to think about it is: You have to deal with 3–4 terrible nights and then the problem is gone. Your child, you, and other kids in the home will be all able to go to sleep without any trouble. You will realize that all of this hard work paid off and that balance is restored in your home.

Several times I have worked with two-parent families in which one parent is on board with using this approach and the other parent is not. I will then defer to the parent who doesn't favor this approach and ask them to come up with a plan on how we can challenge the sleep problem; most of the time, we end up doing the plan by the next week! Sometimes one parent will leave the house for 3–5 nights (oftentimes with siblings), which has been successful for many families. Other times, one parent really needs the support of the other, and a "double team" or "we mean business" in a united front can hold a lot of weight in the process. Regardless of who completes the plan or when, being 100% consistent and predictable in how you will respond to your child's attempt to be with you at bedtime is essential. The plan works, you and your child become better sleepers, and the health of the family improves. Give yourself encouragement that you are doing this for good reasons and that you will have a great outcome. I've never had a parent regret doing this plan or regret getting a child to sleep on his own.

12

Parenting Your Anxious Child

Adopting a Resilience Mindset

A s your child's parent, you are in a unique position to influence him and his process of overcoming his fears. By mastering the best approach to supporting your child and encouraging him on the path of betterment, you can bring him forward in outstanding ways. This chapter will provide guidance on what to do and what to say in response to your child's anxiety; it will also focus on the larger picture: how to support your child's confidence, give him the right messages that will protect him from anxiety in the future, and help to make him resilient. This chapter is about mastering how to be a positive influence on him and his anxiety.

Parenting is a tough job for everyone; effective parents spend their time learning new skills and applying them, and are constantly adapting to their child's developmental stage. Parenting a child with anxiety adds another layer of toughness and requires an additional set of skills. Sometimes parents who struggled with discipline will struggle more in parenting around anxiety, as both share the skill of setting firm boundaries and being consistent; likewise, parents who have mastered a discipline approach that works, one that involves letting their child tolerate disappointment and employs good boundary-setting will have a head start on being able to successfully parent their anxious child. For example, parents who previously were able to sleep train and get their child to sleep on their own (e.g., "you cannot sleep in our bed—we need to get you back in your bed") will likely be more natural at not accommodating the anxiety, as they have had some practice at successfully not accommodating in the past. Parents who have adopted the "permissive" type of parenting (high warmth, low demand) will have more work to do than those who were already employing "authoritative" parenting (high warmth, high demand; Baumrind, 1991). The important thing is to know what skills you need to learn, what you can draw on from past success, or what you need to do differently this time. Either way, helping your child overcome his anxiety will make you a better parent overall. Effective parents will learn these skills (even if they hadn't had practice before), will learn how to be the best parent to an anxious child, and will become a crucial part of treatment success.

Parents who practice the relaxation strategies, review the self-talk cards, and challenge thinking errors have a better result for their child. Parents who make the exposures happen by planning them out and practicing them over and over will also have a better result for their child. Learning how to respond when your child's anxiety rises (as it will when listening to worry loop recordings and practicing steps on the ladder) is essential. Coaching her on how to work through the anxiety and how to stick with it and tolerate the discomfort (rather than avoiding it), and then praising her for her efforts is the equation for success.

Warm, loving parents unintentionally reinforce a child's fear by accommodating it. By changing the environment or doing things differently or facilitating avoidance (all forms of accommodation), anxiety becomes stronger and children miss the opportunity to learn how to be resilient and handle what comes their way. Providing reassurance is a problem because first of all, it doesn't work, and second of all, it gives more power to anxiety and anxious thoughts (e.g., the child thinks "if Mom is spending so much time telling me it's safe in our house, maybe it really isn't"—in other words, if she is working so hard to make me feel safe, then there must be a threat!). **Reassurance validates the anxiety and makes your child more anxious**. Although parents do not cause anxiety, the way they respond to the anxiety absolutely can influence it, in either good or bad ways. The following is a list of replacement responses to use when your child seeks reassurance from you, or wants you to make accommodations on behalf of her anxiety.

Sample parental responses that encourage challenging the anxiety and replace accommodating it include:

- ▶ "I see how hard this is for you. I know you can talk back to the anxiety."
- ▶ "If you are scared, this is your chance to practice being brave. You can only practice being brave when you are scared."
- ▶ "It's only the anxiety talking. What can you say back?"
- ▶ "I know that you want me to answer your questions, but I can't talk to the anxiety. I can talk to you, but not the anxiety."
- ▶ "What can you do to calm down and relax?"
- ▶ "I see you are having a hard time calming down right now. Let's do your breathing and read your cards to help."
- ▶ "Even though it may not feel like it, you can handle this."
- ▶ "I read in that anxiety book for kids that if I feed into your anxiety, I will make it worse. I have to work really hard and not give into your anxiety. I cannot reassure you (or do the rituals) anymore."

I fully recognize that it is a whole lot easier for me to write this list than it is for you to actually say these things to your child. I know these statements may feel foreign or contrived, but I assure you that every parent who has used this list has put a stop to accommodating the anxiety and their child has benefitted. I have had kids say to me, "Ugh, my dad keeps listening to you and he won't budge. It's so annoying." My response to this is very positive: "I'm so happy to hear this! Your dad is doing his job well and you should really congratulate him on helping you" (very few kids actually do give such congratulations to their parents, by the way, but they get what I'm saying). Being consistent in responding this way is imperative.

When working on the ladder with your child, keep emphasizing how they are on a path of freedom: becoming free from anxiety and its hold on their life. Although it's somewhat contradictory to the spirit of the ladder and this program, sometimes you find yourself in a position in which you have to force your child to face his fears (doing something on his ladder). For example, a middle school girl with a phobia of injections was not going to be allowed to continue to attend school if she didn't receive her vaccines; her parents and therapist essentially forced her to get the shots. They were successful and at the end, she felt better about having been forced; however, during it, it was incredibly challenging for her parents who were not entirely confident that this was the right thing to do with respect to her anxiety. Yet, it was the right thing to do, because what message would the parents send if they said, "You are too afraid of shots and we understand, so you will just not go to school anymore!"? Perhaps you may have to go out of town, which may be a higher step on the ladder for a child with separation anxiety, but you still go even though it's a higher step. Basically, every now and then kids may have to do a step on their ladder they are not prepared for; you can remind them that there is really no such thing as feeling "ready" and sometimes the circumstances are such that facing their fears is necessary. By not accommodating the anxiety and helping your child face his fears and do his ladder, you are modeling how to be proactive, and not reactive, in response to your child's anxiety.

In the *Seven Habits of Highly Successful People*, Stephen Covey (2013) listed "Be Proactive" as the first habit, and went on to explain that proactive people make decisions based on their values, whereas reactive people make decisions based on their feelings. Anxious children, by nature of their anxiety, are reactive. They make decisions whether to do something or not to do something based on their fears. As parents of anxious children, you too, by nature of their anxiety, end up being reactive. Therefore, I recommend the following as the new guiding principle for you, your child, and your family:

> We don't make decision based on anxiety. We don't let anxiety rule our lives, influence our actions, or make decisions for us. We are proactive and make decisions based on what is important to us, based on our values.

When working with kids, I made a handout called "Proactive vs. Reactive" and show them the Seven Habits books (Stephen Covey's son Sean Covey wrote a book for teens, the *Seven Habits of Highly Effective Teens* [2014], which I go through with kids ages 10 and up: specifically, I show the chart on page 51 on proactive and reactive language), and include specific examples of what is proactive and reactive behavior (this is explained in Chapter 7 of your child's book). To explain the terms, I include a generic example of having homework they don't feel like doing: the reactive person says, "I don't feel like doing my homework, so I won't. I'll watch TV instead," while the proactive person says, "I don't feel like doing my homework, but it's important to me to walk into school prepared and show respect to my teachers, so I'll just sit down and get it done." Then I provide personal examples of their anxiety, such as: if you are being reactive you will say, "I'm nervous about going to the sleepover party. What if I get scared and no one will come and get me? It's better not to go, so I won't," while the proactive person says, "I'm nervous about going to the sleepover party, but it's important for me to be social and with my friends, so I'll make myself go and face my fears." Notice that even when someone is being proactive, they still recognize the unpleasant feelings or anticipatory anxiety, but they don't let it organize them or influence their behavior.

You can encourage your child by cuing them to be proactive ("this is a time you can practice being proactive") and also giving them the following proactive-themed self-talk cards:

- ▶ What would someone who is proactive do in this situation?
- ▶ What is the proactive thing to do here?
- ▶ What are my values? I need my behavior to reflect what is truly important to me, not how I feel about the situation (which is being reactive).
- ▶ Think about other times when I've been proactive.
- ▶ I cannot react to the anxiety and let it control my life.

Also, modeling being proactive and putting words to it can really help influence your child. For example, you can say out loud, "There is so much to do today, so many errands, and I just really feel like resting and watching a movie. But, I know it's important to get it all done so let's get going," and then later you can highlight how it paid off to be driven by your values: "I'm so happy it was such a productive day. I've never regretted getting my errands done!" Using your own style, articulating how there are times when you do what needs to get done, even if you don't feel like it (because you act on your values, not your feelings) can offer great modeling.

Being proactive is part of fostering resilience, just like facing one's fears fosters resilience. Resilience is not letting obstacles stand in our way and knowing that no matter what comes our way, we can handle it. Coaching your child on how to problem-solve and not be defeated by obstacles, and to challenge thinking errors that stand in the way (often all-or-nothing thinking or shoulds) builds resilience.

The goal of parenting is to raise an independent, self-sufficient adult. Fostering confidence so they have strong self-esteem and raising them to be resilient supports this goal. In order to be confident and happy, children need to know that they can tolerate discomfort and handle disappointment. That's why giving positive messages about failure is so important. We are designed to have failure: Everyone fails, everyone great fails, every successful person has failed. What matters is how we react to failing, losing, or coming up short. How we respond to making mistakes and failing is more of a reflection of who we are than the fact that we made the mistake or failed at something. I see a lot of perfectionistic kids who are anxious about grades, getting into the "best" colleges, and so on; similarly I give them the message that who they are matters more than where they go to school. When Frank Bruni's book *Where You Go Is Not Who You'll Be: An Antidote to the College Admissions Mania* came out, I started recommending it at every talk I gave to parents at schools. I was relieved by the release of his book, as it echoed exactly how I felt and what I wanted kids and their parents to learn.

A related topic is making sure your child manages stress well, has down time to relax and enjoy life, and is balanced. Creating a good work-life balance is key. Parents need to model this balance. You can work, be a vested parent, be social, and have interests, but they need to be balanced and the more you model going through life in a calm and graceful way, the better the image of adulthood you are projecting for your kids.

Parents who are anxious and/or stressed tend to model being reactive and make thinking errors similar to their kids. The research on Parental Anxiety Management (PAM) shows that children whose parents received training to learn how to manage their own anxiety had better treatment outcomes, *regardless* of if their parents had anxiety or not (Cobham, Dadds, Spence, & McDermott, 2010). This means that everyone wins when they learn how to manage stress and anxiety.

Finally, while many parents can identify with being anxious, some struggle to understand it. They look at their child's anxious reaction and think, "What's the big deal? What's so scary about (a dog, a sleepover, etc.)?" Having and showing empathy for your child and her struggle with anxiety is key. It's crucial that your child feels understood by you, and that even if you don't have firsthand experience with anxiety yourself, you can see and acknowledge her struggle and can validate the challenge of overcoming it. This "mirroring" of her experience will help her feel more confidence in facing her fears and completing this program. Essentially, this is how you become her most supportive team member! Moreover, this empathy will make her achievement of overcoming the anxiety all the more meaningful.

References

American Psychiatric Association. (2013). *Diagnostic and statistical manual of mental disorders* (5th ed.). Washington, DC: Author.

Anxiety Disorder Association of America. (n.d.). *Living and thriving: Children and teens.* Retrieved from http://www.adaa.org/living-with-anxiety/children

Association for Behavioral and Cognitive Therapies. (n.d.). *Treatment options: CBT or medication?* Retrieved from http://www.abct.org/information/?m=minformation&fa=_CBT_Or_Medication

Barlow, D. (2004). Psychological treatments. *American Psychologist, 59,* 869–878.

Baumrind, D. (1971). Current patterns of parental authority. *Developmental Psychology Monograph, 4*(1, Pt.2), 1–103.

Baumrind, D. (1991). The influence of parenting style on adolescent competence and substance use. *Journal of Early Adolescence, 11,* 56–95.

CHADD. (n.d.). *Coexisting symptoms.* Retrieved from http://www.chadd.org/Understanding-ADHD/About-ADHD/Coexisting-Conditions.aspx

Christophersen, E. R., & Mortweet, S. L. (2001). *Treatments that work with children: Empirically supported strategies for managing childhood problems.* Washington, DC: American Psychological Association.

Cobham, V. E., Dadds, M. R., Spence, S. H., & McDermott, B. (2010). Parental anxiety in the treatment of childhood anxiety: A different story three years later. *Journal of Clinical Child & Adolescent Psychology, 39,* 410–420.

Covey, S. (2013). *The 7 habits of highly effective people: Powerful lessons in personal change.* New York, NY: Simon & Schuster.

Covey, S. (2014). *The 7 habits of highly effective teens* (Updated ed.). New York, NY: Simon & Schuster.

Dweck, C. (2006). *Mindset: The new psychology of success.* New York, NY: Random House.

Goel, N., Rao, H., Durmer, J. S., & Dinges, D. F. (2009). Neurocognitive consequences of sleep deprivation. *Seminars in Neurology, 29,* 320–339.

Hollon, S. D., Stewart, M. O., & Strunk, D. (2006). Enduring effects for cognitive behavior therapy in the treatment of depression and anxiety. *Annual Review of Psychology, 57,* 285–315.

Hyman, B. M., & Pedrick, C. (2005). *The OCD workbook: Your guide to breaking free from obsessive-compulsive disorder* (2nd ed.). Oakland, CA: New Harbinger.

Jensen, P. S., Hinshaw, S. P., Kraemer, H. C., Lenora, N., Newcorn, J. H., Abikoff, H. B., . . . Vitello, B. (2001). ADHD comorbidity findings from the MTA study: Comparing comorbid subgroups. *Journal of the American Academy of Child & Adolescent Psychiatry, 40,* 147–158.

Kaufman, G., Raphael, L., & Espeland, P. (1999). *Stick up for yourself: Every kid's guide to personal power and positive self-esteem.* Minneapolis, MN: Free Spirit.

Leahy, R. L. (2006). *The worry cure: Seven steps to stop worry from stopping you.* New York, NY: Harmony Books.

Maccoby, E. E., & Martin, J. A. (1983). Socialization in the context of the family: Parent-child interaction. In P. H. Mussen (Ed.) & E. M. Hetherington (Vol. Ed.), *Handbook of child psychology: Vol. 4: Socialization, personality, and social development* (4th ed., pp. 1–101). New York, NY: Wiley.

Mehrabian, A., & Ferris, S. R. (1967). Inference of attitudes from nonverbal communication in two channels. *Journal of Consulting Psychology, 31,* 248–252.

Merikangas, K. R., He, J., Burstein, M., Swanson, S. A., Avenevoli, S., Cui, L., . . . Swendsen, J. (n.d.). *Any anxiety disorder among children.* Retrieved from http://www.nimh.nih.gov/health/statistics/prevalence/any-anxiety-disorder-among-children.shtml

Otte, C. (2011). Cognitive behavioral therapy in anxiety disorders: current state of the evidence. *Dialogues in Clinical Neuroscience, 13,* 413–421.

Price, A. M. H., Wake, M., Ukomunne, O. C., & Hiscock., H. (2012). Five-year follow-up of harms and benefits of behavioral infant sleep intervention: Randomized trial. *Pediatrics, 130,* 643–651.

Sburlati, E. S., Lyneham, H. J., Schniering, C. A., & Rapee, R. M. (Eds.). (2014). *Evidence-based CBT for anxiety and depression in children and adolescents: A competencies based approach.* Chichester, England: Wiley Blackwell.

Sells, S. P. (2002). *Parenting your out-of-control teenager: 7 steps to reestablish authority and reclaim love.* New York, NY: St. Martin's Griffin.

Storch, E. A., Geffken, G. R., Merlo, L. J., Jacob, M. L., Murphy, T. K., Goodman, W. K., . . . Grabill, K. (2007). Family accommodation in pediatric obsessive-compulsive disorder. *Journal of Clinical Child & Adolescent Psychology, 36,* 207–216.

Walkup, J. T., Albano, A. M., Piacentini, J., Birmaher, B., Compton, S. N., Sherrill, J. T., . . . Kendall, P. C. (2008). Cognitive behavioral therapy, sertraline, or a combination in childhood anxiety. *New England Journal of Medicine, 359,* 2753–2766.

Wells, A. (2011). *Metacognitive therapy for anxiety and depression.* New York, NY: Guilford Press.

Wilson, R. R. (2003). *Facing panic: Self-help for people with panic attacks.* Silver Spring, MD: Anxiety Disorders Association of America.

Wolk, C. B., Kendall, P. C., & Beidas, R. S. (2015). Cognitive-behavioral therapy for child anxiety confers long-term protection from suicidality. *Journal of the American Academy of Child & Adolescent Psychiatry, 54,* 175–179.

Resources for Parents

Recommended Books and Articles
for Parents and Professionals

General Anxiety

Bourne, E. J. (2015). *The anxiety & phobia workbook* (6th ed.). Oakland, CA: New Harbinger.

Leahy, R. L. (2006). *The worry cure: Seven steps to stop worry from stopping you.* New York, NY: Harmony Books.

Wilson, R., & Lyons, L. (2013). *Anxious kids, anxious parents: 7 ways to stop the worry cycle and raise courageous and independent children.* Deerfield Beach, FL: HCI Publishing.

Separation Anxiety

Eisen, A. R., & Engler, L. B. (2006). *Helping your child overcome separation anxiety or school refusal: A step-by-step guide for parents.* Oakland, CA: New Harbinger.

Social Anxiety

Antony, M. M., & Swinson, R. P. (2008). *The shyness and social anxiety workbook: Proven step-by-step techniques for overcoming your fears* (2nd ed.). Oakland, CA: New Harbinger.

OCD

Chansky, T. E. (2001). *Freeing your child from obsessive-compulsive disorder: A powerful, practical program for parents of children and adolescents.* Danvers, MA: Harmony.

Hyman, B. M., & Pedrick, C. (2010). *The OCD workbook: Your guide to breaking free from obsessive-compulsive disorder* (3rd ed.). Oakland, CA: New Harbinger.

Panic Attacks

Wilson, R. R. (2003). *Facing panic: Self-help for people with panic attacks.* Silver Spring, MD: Anxiety Disorders Association of America.

Perfectionism

Adelson, J. L., & Wilson, H. E. (2009). *Letting go of perfect: Overcoming perfectionism in kids.* Waco, TX: Prufrock Press.

Antony, M. M., & Swinson, R. P. (2009). *When perfect isn't good enough: Strategies for coping with perfectionism* (2nd ed.). Oakland, CA: New Harbinger.

Health Anxiety

Taylor, S., & Asmundson, G. J. G. (2004). *Treating health anxiety: A cognitive-behavioral approach.* New York, NY: Guilford Press.

Hair Pulling

Keuthen, N. J., Stein, D. J., & Christenson, G. A. (2001). *Help for hair pullers: Understanding and coping with trichotillomania.* Oakland, CA: New Harbinger.

Mouton-Odum, S., & Golomb, R. G. G. (2013). *A parent guide to hair pulling disorder: Effective parenting strategies for children with trichotillomania.* Goldum Publishing.

Pentzel, F. (2003). *The hair-pulling problem: A complete guide to trichotillomania.* New York, NY: Oxford University Press.

Parenting and Discipline (School Refusal)

Baumrind, D. (1991). The influence of parenting style on adolescent competence and substance use. *Journal of Early Adolescence, 11,* 56–95.

Brooks, R., & Goldstein, S. (2002). *Raising resilient children: Fostering strength, hope, and optimism in your child.* New York, NY: McGraw-Hill.

Bruni, F. (2015). *Where you go is not who you'll be: An antidote to the college admissions mania.* New York, NY: Grand Central Publishing.

Dweck, C. (2006). *Mindset: The new psychology of success.* New York, NY: Random House.

Kazdin, A. E. (2009). *The Kazdin Method for parenting the defiant child.* New York, NY: Mariner.

Maccoby, E. E., & Martin, J. A. (1983). Socialization in the context of the family: Parent-child interaction. In P. H. Mussen (Ed.) & E. M. Hetherington (Vol. Ed.), *Handbook of child psychology: Vol. 4: Socialization, personality, and social development* (4th ed., pp. 1–101). New York, NY: Wiley.

Phelan, T. W. (2016). *1-2-3 magic: Effective discipline for children 2–12* (6th ed.). Naperville, IL: Sourcebooks.

Sells, S. P. (2002). *Parenting your out-of-control teenager: 7 steps to reestablish authority and reclaim love.* New York, NY: St. Martin's Griffin.

Siegel, D., & Hartzell, M. (2013). *Parenting from the inside out: How a deeper self-understanding can help you raise children who thrive* (10th anniversary ed.). New York, NY: Tarcher/Penguin.

Walsh, D. (2007). *No: Why kids—of all ages—need to hear it and ways parents can say it.* New York, NY: Free Press.

Selective Mutism

McHolm, A. E., Cunningham, C. E., & Vanier, M. K. (2005). *Helping your child with selective mutism: Practical steps to overcome a fear of speaking.* Oakland, CA: New Harbinger.

Bedwetting

Bennett, H. J. (2015). *Waking up dry: A guide to help children overcome bedwetting* (2nd ed.). Elk Grove Village, IL: American Academy of Pediatrics.

Sensory Processing Disorder

Gibbs, V., & Whitney, R. (2013). *Raising kids with sensory processing disorders: A week-by-week guide to solving everyday sensory issues.* Waco, TX: Prufrock Press.

Kranowitz, C. S. (2006). *The out-of-sync child: Recognizing and coping with sensory processing disorder* (2nd ed.). New York, NY: Perigee.

Medication

Wilens, T. (2016). *Straight talk about psychiatric medications for kids* (4th ed.). New York, NY: Guilford Press.

Nutrition and Dietary

Fuhrman, J. (2006). *Disease-proof your child: Feeding kids right.* New York, NY: St. Martin's Press.

Perlmutter, D. (2013). *Grain brain: The surprising truth about wheat, carbs, and sugar—Your brain's silent killers.* New York, NY: Little, Brown, & Company.

Mindfulness and Meditation and Yoga

NurrieSteams, M. (2010). *Yoga for anxiety: Meditations and practices for calming the body and mind.* Oakland, CA: New Harbinger.

Singer, M.A. (2007). *The untethered soul: The journey beyond yourself.* Oakland, CA: New Harbinger.

Snel, E. (2013). *Sitting still like a frog: Mindfulness exercises for kids (and their parents).* Boston, MA: Shambhala Publications.

Recommended Books for Children

Covey, S. (2014). *The 7 habits of highly effective teens.* New York, NY: Touchstone.

Crist, J. J. (2004). *What to do when you're scared and worried: A guide for kids.* Minneapolis, MN: Free Spirit.

Flanagan, E. (2014). *Ten turtles on Tuesday: A story for children about obsessive compulsive disorder.* Washington, DC: Magination Press.

Golomb, R. G., & Vavrichek, S. M. (2000). *The hair pulling "habit" and you: How to solve the trichotillomania puzzle* (Rev. ed.). Silver Spring, MD: Writers Cooperative of Greater Washington.

Guber, T., & Kalish, L. (2005). *Yoga pretzels.* Cambridge, MA: Barefoot Books. (Yoga cards)

Huebner, D. (2007). *What to do when your brain gets stuck: A kid's guide to overcoming OCD.* Washington, DC: Magination Press.

Kaufman, G., Raphael, L., & Espeland, P. (1999). *Stick up for yourself: Every kid's guide to personal power and positive self-esteem.* Minneapolis, MN: Free Spirit.

Kendall, P. C. (2006). *Coping cat workbook* (2nd ed.). Ardmore, PA: Workbook Publishing.

Wagner, A. P., & Jutton, P. A., (2013). *Up and down the worry hill: A children's book about obsessive-compulsive disorder and its treatment.* Rochester, NY: Lighthouse Press.

Recommended CDs

Alvord, M., Zucker, B., & Alvord, B. (2011). *Relaxation and self-regulation techniques for children and teens: Mastering the mind-body connection* [Audio CD]. Champaign, IL: Research Press.

Charlesworth, E. A. (2002). *Scanning relaxation* [Audio CD]. Champaign, IL: Research Press.

Lite, L. (2006). *Indigo dreams: Relaxation and stress management bedtime stories for children, improve sleep, manage stress and anxiety* [Audio CD]. Marietta, GA: Lite Books.

Recommended Apps

- ▶ Calm.com
- ▶ CBT Tools for Kids
- ▶ Headspace
- ▶ Insight Timer

Organizations

American Psychological Association (APA)
750 First Street, NE
Washington, DC 20002
800-374-2721
http://www.apa.org
http://www.apa.org/helpcenter

The Anxiety Disorders Association of America (ADAA)
8701 Georgia Avenue, Suite 412
Silver Spring, MD 20910
240-485-1001
http://www.adaa.org

Association for Behavioral and Cognitive Therapies (ABCT)

305 7th Avenue, 16th Fl.
New York, NY 10001
212-647-1890
http://www.abct.org

The Child Anxiety Network

http://www.childanxiety.net

National Alliance on Mental Illness (NAMI)

3803 N. Fairfax Drive, Suite 100
Arlington, VA 22203
800-950-6264
http://www.nami.org

National Institute of Mental Health (NIMH)

Science Writing, Press, and Dissemination Branch
6001 Executive Boulevard, Room 6200, MSC 9663
Bethesda, MD 20892
866-615-6464
http://www.nimh.nih.gov

International OCD Foundation (IOCDF)

P.O. Box 961029
Boston, MA 02196
617-973-5801
http://www.ocfoundation.org

The TLC Foundation for Body-Focused Repetitive Behaviors (formerly Trichotillomania Learning Center, Inc.)

716 Soquel Ave., Suite A
Santa Cruz, CA 95062
831-457-1004
http://www.bfrb.org

Appendix A

Overview of the Program

This page provides an overview of the program and allows you and your child to check off when each of the chapters and exercises are completed.

Chapter	Topic	☑ Done
Chapter 1	Anxiety: What It Is and What To Do About It Exercise: Fill in the Bubbles	
Chapter 2	Making Your Team and Team Goals Exercise: Making Your Team and Team Goals	
Chapter 3	Relaxing the Body Exercise: Practice Relaxation	
Chapter 4	Conquer Your Worries Exercise: Self-Talk Note Cards and Worry Tapes	
Chapter 5	Changing Your Thoughts Exercise: Identify and Replace Thinking Errors	
Chapter 6	Changing Your Behaviors: Facing Your Fears Exercise: Facing Your Fears	
Chapter 7	Keep Facing Your Fears and Build Confidence Exercise: Finish Your Ladder	
Chapter 8	Lessons Learned: Celebrate Yourself Exercise: Party and Certificate	

(The parent's guide has four additional chapters: Chapter 9: Motivating Your Child; Chapter 10: Special Sections; Chapter 11: Anxiety at Bedtime: Improving Sleep Behavior; and Chapter 12: Parenting Your Anxious Child: Adopting a Resilience Mindset.)

Appendix B

Thinking Errors Quick Reference Page

- *Catastrophizing:* visualizing disaster; thinking that the worst thing is going to happen and feeling like you wouldn't be able to handle it; asking "What if . . ."
- *All-or-Nothing:* thinking in extremes, things are either perfect or a failure; there is no middle ground—it's either one extreme or another; thinking in an inflexible way
- *Filtering:* focusing on the negative parts of a situation while ignoring the positive parts; catching all the bad parts and forgetting about the good parts
- *Magnifying:* making something seem bigger and worse than it really is; turning up the volume on anything bad
- *Shoulds:* rules that you have about how things should be; using the words "should," "must," and "ought to" to show how things should be
- *Mind Reading:* thinking you know what others are thinking, particularly what they are thinking about you; usually you will think that others are thinking negatively about you
- *Overgeneralization:* taking a single incident and thinking that it will always be this way; something happens once and you think it will always happen this way
- *Personalization:* taking something personally; making it about you when it has nothing to do with you
- *Selective Attention:* paying attention to things that confirm your beliefs about something; ignoring evidence that goes against what you believe about a particular situation
- *Probability Overestimation:* overestimating the likelihood that something bad will happen

About the Author

Bonnie Zucker, Psy.D., is a licensed psychologist with a background and expertise in psychotherapy with children, adolescents, and adults. She received her doctoral degree in clinical psychology from Illinois School of Professional Psychology in Chicago, her master's degree in applied psychology from University of Baltimore, and her bachelor's degree in psychology from The George Washington University.

Dr. Zucker specializes in the treatment of childhood anxiety disorders. Using a cognitive-behavioral (CBT) approach, she has helped hundreds of children become anxiety-free by teaching them coping skills, methods for challenging their faulty thinking, and how to systematically face their fears. Dr. Zucker also integrates a family systems approach in order to teach parents how to most appropriately respond to their child's anxiety disorder.

Dr. Zucker is in private practice in Rockville, MD. She was named one of *Washingtonian* Magazine's Top Therapists in several fields, including CBT, OCD, and phobias. In addition to being active in training mental health professionals on the treatment of anxiety disorders, Dr. Zucker wrote *Take Control of OCD: The Ultimate Guide for Kids With OCD* and *Something Very Sad Happened: A Toddler's Guide to Understanding Death*. She also coauthored *Resilience Builder Program for Children & Adolescents: Enhancing Social Competence & Self Regulation (A Cognitive-Behavioral Group Approach)*, *Relaxation & Self-Regulation Techniques for Children & Teens: Mastering the Mind-Body Connection* (Audio CD), and *Relaxation & Wellness Techniques: Mastering the Mind-Body Connection* (Audio CD).

Anxiety-Free Kids

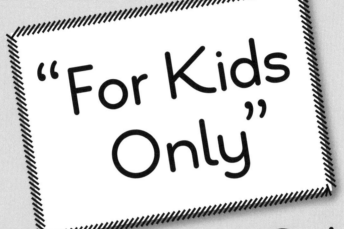

"For Kids Only"

Companion Guide

Bonnie Zucker, Psy.D.

(That means she's a psychologist!)

Table of Contents

Welcome to *Anxiety-Free Kids* and Dr. Zucker's
"For Kids Only" Companion Guide v

Introduction 1

CHAPTER 1
Anxiety: *What It Is and What to Do About It* 3

CHAPTER 2
Making Your Team and Team Goals 13

CHAPTER 3
Relaxing the Body 21

CHAPTER 4
Conquer Your Worries 37

CHAPTER 5
Changing Your Thoughts 49

CHAPTER 6
Changing Your Behaviors: *Facing Your Fears* 67

CHAPTER 7
Keep Facing Your Fears and Build Confidence 73

CHAPTER 8
Lessons Learned: *Celebrate Yourself* 83

Appendix A: *Overview of the Program* 89

Appendix B: *Thinking Errors Quick Reference Page* 91

Welcome to *Anxiety-Free Kids* and Dr. Zucker's "For Kids Only" Companion Guide

WELCOME to Dr. Zucker's "For Kids Only" Companion Guide to the book *Anxiety-Free Kids*, second edition! My name is Dr. Bonnie Zucker and I am a type of doctor called a *psychologist*. My job is to work with kids just like you who are having a hard time with worries and fears and help them feel better. The best thing I do to help them is to teach them how to *face their fears*. I'll talk more about this later and explain what it means. Kids usually come to see me once a week, and we talk about what makes them feel scared (it's called *therapy*). During therapy, we try to come up with ways to overcome these fears. Their parent also comes in at the end of the meeting to learn how to help them deal with being afraid and worrying. We all work together as a team.

This book will help you make your own team to help you face your fears.

Your parent (or someone else who cares for you a lot) got this book for you to help you deal with times when you worry or feel scared. Worrying and being scared also is called *anxiety*. When someone has anxiety or feels scared a lot, it is not his fault, and he shouldn't feel embarrassed or ashamed. A lot of kids experience the same anxiety, but they just might not talk about it. But, because feeling this way can make kids feel really bad at times, and can keep them from doing things they would like to be able to do, it is a good idea to work on these feelings and make them better. So this is what this book is all about—helping you to feel better! Feeling better also usually means feeling stronger, and other kids who learn how to deal with their anxiety say that they feel more sure of them-selves. By becoming a "master" of your anxiety, you will no longer have to be afraid or worry about bad things happening. You will no longer have to avoid doing certain things.

The information in this book is the same information I talk about with kids who meet with me in my office. Maybe you already meet with a psychologist like me, or maybe you don't. Either way, you should feel very proud of yourself for starting this program—helping yourself get better is a very grown-up thing to do!

Good luck,
Dr. Bonnie Zucker

Introduction

BEFORE we get started, let me tell you a little about how this book works. Your parent (or whoever gave this book to you) is going to be reading his or her own book that goes along with your book (it's called a *companion book*). The chapters are matched up with one another so that your parent is always reading about the same thing as you. For example, in this book, Chapter 1 is all about anxiety. In your parent's book, Chapter 1 also is about anxiety.

At the end of each chapter, there are exercises for you and your parent to do together. Sometimes these will involve questions to answer together, or suggestions on what to talk about, or you may be asked to do a short activity. Whatever it is, you will work on it with your parent. Your parent's book will tell her about these exercises, as well, and your parent will read about ways she can help you complete them. The exercises are very important and often will be fun to do!

Two last things you should know. First, while I realize that many kids are raised by stepparents, grandparents, aunts and uncles, and other loving adults, I will use words like "parents," "mom," and "dad" to describe the person who is completing this program with you. If you are one of these kids, just know that when you see me talk about your parent, mom, or dad, I mean the person who gave you this book. Whoever that person is cares about you a lot and wants to help you overcome your anxiety and feel better. Second, I will use different girls' and boys' names throughout the book as examples. This is because both girls and boys have worries and anxiety.

OK, let's get started!

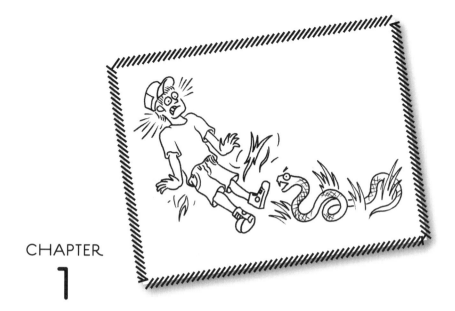

CHAPTER

1

Anxiety

What It Is and What to Do About It

WHEN you are feeling nervous, worried, scared, or afraid, this is called *anxiety*, or feeling anxious. The opposite of feeling anxious is feeling relaxed. Everyone—kids and adults—feels nervous from time to time. Sometimes something will happen to make you feel anxious, such as when you are in a store and you cannot find your mom or dad, when you have to get a shot at the doctor's office, or when the electricity goes out and you're alone in your room. Other times, it comes out of the blue, and you just feel nervous for no reason. When this happens, you may start to worry about bad things happening. These worries usually make you feel more scared and nervous. Kids who feel scared or nervous much of the time often begin to feel bad about themselves, and worry about how well they can handle things. When you are not sure if you are able to handle something, this is called *self-doubt*. It is common to feel this way and you should not feel bad about yourself because you have anxiety and worries.

Anxiety becomes a concern when it starts to cause problems in your everyday life. For example, if your worries are preventing you from going to school, birthday parties, sleepovers, or sleeping alone at night, then it is causing a problem. If you get a lot of stomachaches or headaches, or feel like you don't have the energy to do things, it might be because of anxiety. Also, if you have trouble concentrating at school because you are focusing on your worries, then anxiety is causing a problem for you.

Let me give you some examples of kids who have anxiety:

► When James was 6 years old, he was in his backyard helping his father pull weeds from the garden. As he pulled out one very big weed, a garden snake jumped out at him and landed right on his stomach before it fell to the ground and glided away. Even though James was not hurt by the snake at all, after this happened, James became afraid of snakes. He began to worry about seeing another snake. Whenever he was in his backyard, he would be on guard looking for snakes. Sometimes, he would hear an animal moving in the bushes and he would run away, fearing that it was a snake in there. As he grew up, James's fear grew and grew. When he watched a scene from one of the *Harry Potter* movies that had a snake in it, he became very scared, even though the friends he was watching it with were not scared. James even refused to go to his friend's house because his friend had a pet snake. Sometimes James would feel sick to his stomach just thinking of snakes. When he turned 12, he came to therapy to learn ways to get over his fear of snakes. In therapy, he learned that he had what is called a *phobia* of snakes.

▶ Billy was a very smart 9-year-old with a great imagination. He loved to design creative games, and was always happy when he worked on his games. Even though he was one of the smartest kids in his class, Billy took a very long time to do writing assignments at school because he had a learning disability. Some of his teachers did not understand about his learning disability, and would punish him for not having all of his work done. Sometimes, his teacher even made him stay in from recess to finish his work. This made Billy feel uncomfortable and embarrassed. He started to worry about getting in trouble and having to stay back during recess. He worried so much that his muscles became all tense, he couldn't sleep at night, and he even got stomachaches and headaches. Because he felt so nervous about writing and about getting in trouble if he didn't get all of his work done, Billy would daydream and couldn't focus on his work. He worried so much that it was hard for him to concentrate. Sometimes he would be so worried that he would not want to go to school. Billy came to therapy and learned that he had what is called *generalized anxiety.*

▶ Ten-year-old Ruth spent a lot of time worrying that she would get sick. She worried that she would get sick by getting germs from others. Whenever she was at a sleepover or a party, Ruth refused to eat food from bowls that others had touched. She never ate anything homemade, especially homemade cookies or brownies, or anything from the school cafeteria. Ruth had a very hard time using public bathrooms; it was so uncomfortable for her, that she often "held it" until she got home. When she did use public bathrooms, she did her best not to touch anything there. She would flush the toilet with her foot so she didn't have to touch the flusher, and she used her sleeve to touch the faucet and door handles so she wouldn't have to touch it with her hands. If Ruth accidentally touched anything in the bathroom, even the walls of the stall, she would insist that her mother wash her clothes immediately once they got home. She wanted her mom to wash everything twice, to make sure the germs were gone. Even though she didn't really know why she was so afraid of germs, sometimes she would become so upset about getting germs on her, that she would stay at home in her room all day. Ruth's parents brought her to therapy and she learned that she had a type of anxiety called *obsessive-compulsive disorder.*

James, Billy, and Ruth all had anxiety that caused problems in their lives. All of their worries and fears were very upsetting for them, and got in the way of doing normal, everyday things, like going into the backyard, going to school, using public bathrooms, and even eating homemade cookies! Their anxiety and fears went past "normal" amounts, which they all learned was why they had to get help for their anxiety problems. All three of them got help and all three of them got over their anxiety. James, Billy, and Ruth no longer have problems with anxiety. You'll hear more about them and how they did it later in this book.

Now let me teach you the three parts of anxiety: body, thoughts, and behavior. (See Figure 1.)

Anxiety comes out in three ways: in our bodies, our thoughts, and the way we act (our behavior). In order to understand anxiety, we need to understand the three parts of it, and we also need to learn how to make each part better. Let's go through each one.

Body

Our bodies have a reaction when we feel anxious. Different kids have different reactions, but the most common are:

- ▶ fast heartbeat;
- ▶ sweating or sweaty palms;

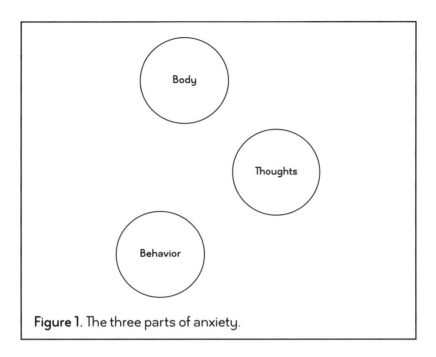

Figure 1. The three parts of anxiety.

- ▶ difficulty breathing (shallow, fast breathing);
- ▶ tense muscles;
- ▶ restlessness;
- ▶ feeling like it's hard to swallow or you are going to choke;
- ▶ stomachaches;
- ▶ headaches;
- ▶ feeling dizzy;
- ▶ shaking; and
- ▶ feeling detached from your body.

Thoughts

When we feel anxious, we usually worry. Worry is a type of thought (for example, we think about scary things happening). Many people worry about bad things happening to them, or to someone they love. Others worry that they won't do well, like on a test, or that other kids or parents won't like them. We also might make "thinking mistakes" or "thinking errors," which are very common. These thoughts make the anxiety worse. You will learn more about thinking mistakes in Chapter 5. Also, we have negative self-talk, which involves saying things to ourselves (usually not out loud) that actually make the anxiety worse. Here are some examples of each:

- ▶ "What if something bad happens to my mom or dad when they go out tonight?" (worry)
- ▶ "What if I fail the test tomorrow?" (worry)
- ▶ "Other kids will laugh at me if I raise my hand and give the wrong answer." (thinking mistake)
- ▶ "I should get all A's in school. If I get a B, it means I am a failure." (thinking mistake)
- ▶ "I can't do this. I will only feel better if I go home right now." (negative self-talk)
- ▶ "I'm so scared, this is terrible." (negative self-talk)

Behavior

The most common behavior or action linked with anxiety and fears is avoidance. Avoidance means you don't do the thing you are afraid of or you stay away from the thing that makes you feel scared. For example, if you are afraid of dogs, you will not go near them. You may refuse to go to a friend's house if he has a dog, or you may leave a park if there are dogs around. If you are afraid when your parents leave the house, you will try to make them stay and not leave. If you are afraid of talking to other kids at school or of raising your hand and talking in front of the class, you will not do these things. Other common anxious or nervous behaviors include: reassurance-seeking (this is a fancy way of saying that you get others, usually your parents, to tell you things that make you feel better), fidgeting or being restless (for example, moving around a lot, not being able to sit still), picking or pulling (for example, picking at your nails, pulling your hair), crying, freezing up, and having a meltdown or tantrum.

Now that you've learned more about the three parts of anxiety, let's look at the circles again with more detail (see Figure 2).

What to Do About Anxiety

We have to work on each part in order to best help you with your anxiety or fears. So, now that you know the three parts of anxiety, let me tell you what we're going to do with each part. For your **body**, I am going to teach you (and your parent will help, too) how to take deep, calm relaxing breaths, how to do something called *progressive muscle relaxation* (PMR for short), how to do relaxing imagery, practice mindfulness, and teach you some yoga poses. For your **thoughts**, you will learn positive self-talk, how to know and change your thinking mistakes, and how to conquer (or master) worry. You will learn when your thinking is realistic (likely to come true) and when it is unrealistic (not likely to come true). You also will learn how to feel better, or more confident, about yourself and your ability to handle things. For your **behavior**, you will learn how to face your fears so that you can overcome them and get rid of any nervous behaviors that you do.

Here are the bubbles one last time (see Figure 3).

This may sound like a lot of work, but I promise you three things:

1. It won't be nearly as hard as you think (plus we'll try to make it a little fun).
2. You will have a team to support you (I'm one of the people on your team!).
3. You definitely will feel a lot better by doing this program!

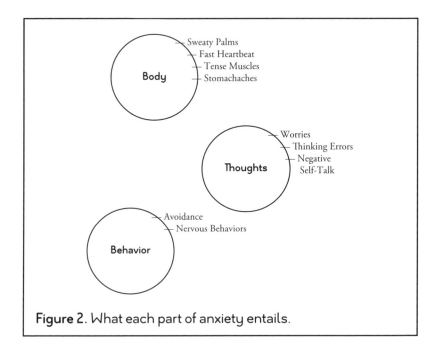

Figure 2. What each part of anxiety entails.

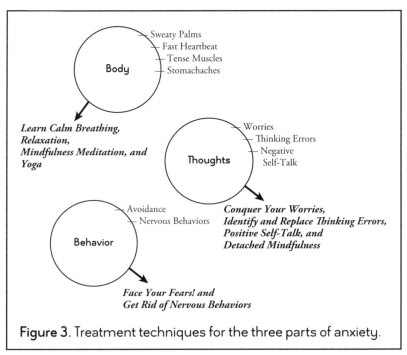

Figure 3. Treatment techniques for the three parts of anxiety.

Chapter 1 EXERCISE

Fill in the Bubbles

Directions: You and your parent will do this together. In each of the bubbles, write in the three parts of anxiety. Next to each part (bubble), write your own examples of your experience with anxiety. For example, you can write down what specific things happen to your body when you are anxious.

(*Hint:* It will end up looking a lot like the one on p. 10.)

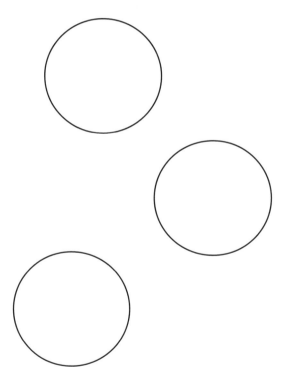

Congratulations on finishing Chapter 1! You should feel very proud of yourself because you have taken the first step in over-coming your anxiety.

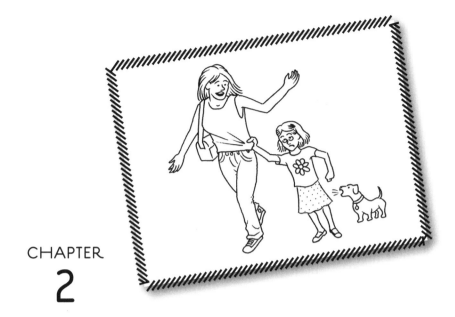

2

Making Your Team and Team Goals

T HIS chapter is shorter to read than the previous one, but the exercise that you and your parent will do is longer than most of the other exercises in this book. The best part is that this exercise is going to be fun. We already talked a little about how important it is to face your fears. Let's talk more about this. As you already learned, when you avoid doing things because you are afraid or nervous to do them, this is called *avoidance behavior* because you are avoiding, or not doing, something. Each time that you don't do something because it makes you feel anxious, *the anxiety wins*. Each time you do something that makes you feel anxious, *you win and the anxiety loses*. It is you against the anxiety (You vs. Anxiety), and I promise you that as you face your fears, you *will* win!

Let me give you an example:

Eight-year-old Thelma was one of the children I worked with in therapy. She was very nice, very smart, and very nervous about being separated from her mom. If her mom went out in the front of the house to take out the trash, Thelma would become anxious—her heart would beat fast, and she would stop doing whatever she was doing to go to the window and watch her mom. Thelma would worry that something bad would happen to her and that she wouldn't come back. Thelma also did not like to be in a different room than her mom, and when her mom would go in another room, Thelma would ask her to sing a song so Thelma would always know where she was. She refused to sleep in her own bed at night even though her mom would try to get her to sleep alone. Thelma would cry and cry and beg her mom to be able to sleep with her. Sometimes, Thelma's mom needed to go out without her and a babysit-ter would come over; this upset Thelma so much that she would get sick and throw up. As soon as her mom would come home, Thelma would feel better.

Thelma had anxiety, and her anxiety was called *separation anx-iety*, which meant that she got very nervous and worried when she was separated from her mom, and worried about bad things hap-pening to her mom. She did her best to *avoid* being separated from her, because this was the thing that made her feel so scared. Each time that Thelma was clinging onto her mom and *avoided* being separated from her, *the anxiety would win and she would lose.* Even though staying near her mom helped her to feel better at the time, it actually made the anxiety much worse overall. Thelma learned that she had to face her fears to overcome them. How did she do it?

Thelma and her team (her mom, sister, and me, Dr. Zucker) worked together to make a list of all of the things that felt scary to her and that were hard to do. Then, Thelma and I put the list in order, from easiest to hardest, and wrote them all on a poster board, in the form of a ladder. Each step on the ladder was one of the things that was hard for her to do. Thelma learned how to relax and take deep breaths, learned that her fears were not realistic (for example, it was perfectly safe for her mom to take out the trash), and learned what to say to herself to help her deal with her scary thoughts and feelings. Thelma also learned that she was making thinking mistakes and worked on correcting them. Finally, she understood that she needed to face her fears, one step (or fear) at a time. She knew that when she was facing her fears, she would have to handle feeling some anxiety, but that the anxiety would go away with time and practice. Most importantly, Thelma was told that she would not have to take any of the steps until she was ready; Thelma would not be forced to face her fears. Instead, Thelma would be encouraged by her team to face her fear—she would be cheered on.

Thelma named her ladder "Climbing to Confidence" because she felt that her separation anxiety made her feel less confident, or sure, about herself. By facing her fears, she would feel more confident. This is what Thelma's ladder looked like:

Climbing to Confidence

(top)	Mom goes out of town without you.
	Go on a sleepover at a friend's house.
	Mom goes out for the day without you.
	Go on a play date at a friend's house.
	Mom goes out for 1 hour, then 2 hours without you.
	Mom goes out for 15 minutes, then 30 minutes without you.
	Sleep in your bed alone one night this week (then 2, 4, 5, and 7 nights).

	You use a public bathroom on your own (without Mom).
	Mom takes the trash out and you stay focused on the TV.
	Mom stays upstairs while you stay downstairs (for 5, 10, 15, and 30 minutes, then for 1 hour).
	Mom goes into other rooms without singing to you.
(bottom)	You stay in living room while Mom is in kitchen (for 5, 10, 15, 20, and 30 minutes).

Thelma practiced her relaxation and deep breathing, read her self-talk note cards, studied the thinking mistakes that she made and how to think more correct or realistic thoughts, and used her tools to master her worry. When she was ready, Thelma took the first step on her ladder: to go in the living room while her mom was in the nearby kitchen. She started slow, doing it for 5 minutes, then did it for longer periods of time—10, 15, 20, and 30 minutes—eventually being able to be in the living room alone for more than an hour! It was not too easy, but it wasn't nearly as hard as she thought it would be. The first time she did it, she called to her mom, who popped her head in the living room and told Thelma that she was facing her fears and doing a fantastic job. She did it again and again, and then it became very easy, and did not cause her to feel scared or nervous at all. By the third time, she did not have to ask her mom to come in, and she learned to feel comfortable being in the living room alone. She was able to relax and enjoy watching TV and reading a book. Then Thelma felt ready to take the second step: Her mom would go into other rooms in the house while Thelma was in the living room or her bedroom, but her mom would not sing to her. Again, she felt nervous and scared the first time they practiced, but it got easier and easier with each practice, and soon Thelma did not feel nervous when her mom left the room. Thelma remembered to do her breathing and read her self-talk note cards. She also told herself that feeling nervous when doing the steps was normal, but that it would get better, and it did!

Like Thelma, you will learn how to face your fears. Like Thelma, you will have a ladder with your own anxieties, and will also form a team. Let's do this now!

EXERCISE

Chapter 2 EXERCISE

Making Your Team and Team Goals

Who Is on Your Team?

Write in the names of the members of your team in the blanks below. You do not have to fill in all of the blanks. Your team will be at least three people: You (the Captain), whoever is reading the parent book (usually Mom or Dad), and me (Dr. Zucker). Other people you can include on your team are your grandparents, sister or brother, babysitter or nanny, pets, and your therapist if you have one. Your team members all will help you to face your fears in different ways. For example, Thelma's dog, Sniffy, was on her team and Sniffy helped her face her fears by being with her in the beginning when she was nervous about her mom leaving her alone in the living room. Sniffy also gave her extra licks when she was happy about doing such a great job in facing her fears.

Your Team:

1. Team Captain: _____
   (your name here)
2. _____
3. _____
4. _____
5. _____
6. _____

Team Goals: Making Your Ladder

You will need the following materials to make your ladder:

- ▶ Blank note cards
- ▶ Poster board (white or another light color)
- ▶ Markers

EXERCISE

- Pen or pencil
- Stickers (stars, happy faces, whatever you want)

To make your ladder:

1. Using note cards and a pen or pencil, write down all of the different things that are hard for you to do or that you avoid doing because of anxiety and worry. Your parent will help you make this list. Write each of these things on a different note card. (Sometimes kids and their parents choose to write it down on a piece of paper before they write it on the note cards; either way works, just as long as each thing is written on a note card.)

2. Use the floor or a table and spread out all of the note cards. Then look carefully at each of the note cards and put them in order from easiest to hardest (your parent will help). The easiest ones will be on the bottom and the hardest ones will be up at the top. Here is what Thelma's note cards looked like before she made them into a ladder:

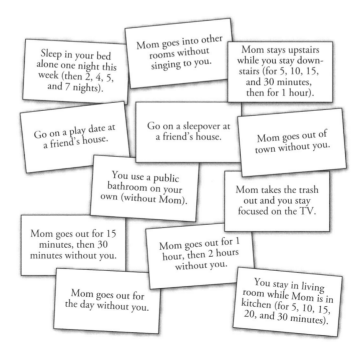

EXERCISE

3. Now count your note cards. How many do you have?

    _____

4. Come up with a title for your ladder. Write the name here:

    _____

Now write the title at the top of the poster board.

5. Use the poster board and markers to draw a great big ladder with steps underneath the place where you wrote the title. The number of steps you draw should be the same as the number of note cards you have. Leave a little space here and there in between some of the steps, just in case you decide to add more things later.

6. Write the steps, from easiest to hardest, on the ladder using the markers.

The stickers will be used once you start doing the steps. We won't begin doing this just yet; first you need to learn some tools (or ways) to deal with your anxious feelings and worries. You first will learn how to help the **body** part of anxiety. In the next chapter, you will learn about relaxation and deep breathing.

Congratulations on making your team and ladder!

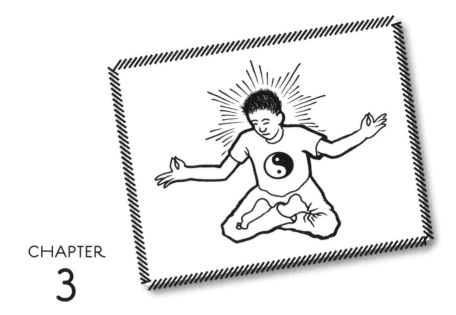

CHAPTER

3

Relaxing the Body

N Chapter 1, you learned that your body has a reaction when you feel anxious or afraid. In this chapter, you will learn how to relax your body and muscles (this chapter is about the body part of the three parts of anxiety). Once you practice the different types of relaxation, you will realize how good it feels to be so relaxed. With practice, you will become a master of relaxation. You also will learn that it is impossible to be relaxed and anxious at the same time. So, if you are feeling anxious and then you use your new skills to relax your body, you will not feel anxious any more.

There are five types of relaxation that we will discuss and practice:

1. calm breathing,
2. progressive muscle relaxation (PMR),

3. relaxing imagery
4. mindfulness meditation, and
5. yoga.

Calm Breathing

When breathing in a calm, relaxed way, you breathe in through your nose and out through your mouth. As you breathe in through your nose, allow the air to travel all the way down to your lower belly. This is the opposite from breathing in an anxious, tense way when your breathing is shallow and the air only goes as far down as the upper part of your chest.

Try doing this: *Breathe in through your nose for the count of 4 and then out through your mouth for the count of 4.* As you do this, try to get the air that you breathe in to go all the way to the bottom of your belly, below your belly button. It helps if you put your hands on this part of your belly and then try to get your hands to move up and down as you breathe in and out. Try not to let any air stop, or get stuck, in the top of your chest; just let the air go in easily through your nose all the way to the bottom of your belly.

Look at Thelma as she learns how to do calm breathing. Notice how her lower belly goes out as she breathes in.

Now *breathe in through your nose for the count of 4, hold the breath for a few seconds, and then slowly breathe out through your mouth for the count of 4.* It also may help to practice doing this when lying down on the floor and putting a yoga block or a book on the top part of your chest (a few inches below your neck); watch how the block (or book) moves up and down when the breath only goes into your upper chest—this is anxious breathing. When we are anxious or nervous, our breath tends to only stay in the "shallow" end of our chest (the upper part), but when we are calm and relaxed, the breath slowly and smoothly goes down to the "deep end" (the lower part of your belly near your belly button), and the upper chest stays still. Practice breathing so the only part that moves up and down is the lower part of your belly.

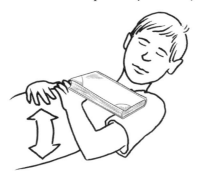

Sometimes kids will have a hard time catching their breath when they are anxious. If this happens to you, try breathing in and out through only one nostril. Let's practice one-nostril breathing: *Hold one of your nostrils closed and close your mouth, then breathe in and out through only one nostril.* Start with the count of 5 (5 in and 5 out), eventually getting up to 10 (10 in and 10 out). When doing one-nostril breathing, don't focus so much on if your upper chest or lower belly is moving, instead focus your attention on slowly breathing in and out through only one nostril. When you do this type of breathing for 5 minutes, you will see how calm and relaxed you can become, just from doing calm breathing!

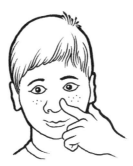

It's very important to know that kids learn calm breathing best when they practice while they are calm; they become masters of calm breathing by learning how to do it when they are already relaxed. This way, you will know what to do when you are anxious—you will know how it feels to do calm breathing.

Progressive Muscle Relaxation (PMR)

PMR is a type of relaxation that involves making your muscles relax by first tightening them up and holding them for the count of 5–10 seconds. You do one section of your body at a time, starting with your hands and going all the way down to your feet. When you do PMR, focus on what it feels like when your muscles are tight and tense and when they are loose and relaxed. OK, let's practice:

1. Start by making tight fists with your hands, imagining that you are squeezing the juice out of a lemon. Hold your fists nice and tight and count to 10. Then let go and shake it out (shake your hands out). Notice how it feels when your muscles are tight and tense versus when they are loose and relaxed.

2. Now pull your arms into your body, next to your ribs. Tighten up your bicep and forearms muscles, but do not make fists or tighten your hands. Hold it for 1, 2, 3, 4, 5, 6, 7, 8, 9, and 10, then let it go and shake it out. Remember to notice what your muscles feel like when they are tense and when they are loose. Sometimes after you loosen them, your muscles will feel a little tingly.

3. Bring your shoulders all the way up toward your ears and tighten them up; this should also make the back of your neck tight. Hold it for the count of 10, then allow your shoulders to drop down toward your hips. As you do this, say the word "Relax" to yourself and also breathe out slowly through your mouth.

4. Now pull your shoulders back and arch your back in toward your chest, trying to get your elbows to touch. Imagine that there is a string connected to your chest and someone is pulling the string up, lifting your chest up toward the ceiling. This will tighten your back. Hold it for a count of 10, then let it go and feel the difference between tension and relaxation.

5. Squeeze and pull your stomach, or abdominal, muscles in toward your spine. Keep it tight for 10 seconds, then let it go.

6. Now squeeze your buttocks muscles (they are important, too!), and hold for 10 seconds, then let go and loosen them up.

7. Stick your legs and feet straight out in front of you and point your toes in toward your chest. This will tighten the muscles in your legs and thighs. Make the muscles as tight as you can and hold for 10 seconds, then let go and allow your legs to gently drop to the ground and relax.

8. Stick your legs and feet straight out in front of you again, but this time point your toes straight out away from you and tighten up the muscles in your legs, thighs, and feet. Try to get it so you feel a little cramping in the bottom of your feet. Hold for 10 seconds, then let go, allowing your legs to gently drop to the floor.

9. Now we will tighten up all of the muscles in your face. Start by clenching your teeth and jaw. Then squish up your nose, lifting it up, and close your eyes and squeeze the muscles around them, and tighten up your forehead. Hold this tightness in your whole face for 10 seconds then let go and relax. Open your mouth a little bit and move your jaw from left to right and then in circles. This will allow the jaw to become even more relaxed.

10. Last step: whole body! You want to go from being a stiff, tight robot to being a loose, relaxed rag doll. Start with

tight fists, then add arms, bring shoulders up to your ears and then pull them back to tighten your back, squeeze your stomach into your spine, tighten your buttocks, put your legs out in front of you with your toes pointing out away from you and cramp up your feet, and tighten your jaw and whole face. Hold for 10 seconds (robot) and then let go (rag doll), loosening every muscle in your body. I could tell if you were a really relaxed rag doll if I tried to lift up your arm and it felt very heavy and loose.

Relaxing Imagery

Relaxing imagery is another type of relaxation, and it is best to first learn and practice it at home or in your therapist's office. You and your parent will do it together as part of the exercise at the end.

Find a comfortable place to sit or lie down. Some kids really like to use pillows, too. If you want to use pillows to get more comfortable, try putting one under your head, another one under your knees, and maybe one under each of your arms. You also may enjoy listening to some relaxing music (with no words) in the background.

Once you are comfortable, I want you to *close your eyes and take a deep breath in through your nose and out through your mouth.* As you breathe in, imagine that you are breathing in clean, relaxing air and as you breathe out, let go of any stress or tension that you are holding onto. Breathing in, you let calm air go all the way down to the bottom of your belly. Breathing out, you let go of the air and your belly becomes flat. With each breath, you feel more and more relaxed. Your parent will read the following script to you, but you can also read over it to help practice getting relaxed.

Imagine that you are standing in a hallway. This is the most beautiful hallway you have ever been in—the floor is cushiony and soft, and the colors that surround you are all of your favorites. The temperature is perfect—cool but not too cool—and you feel a slight breeze on your face. You notice that your body begins to loosen up.

You begin to walk down the hallway and as you do, you feel lighter and lighter. The hallway curves around to the left and then curves around to the right. As you are walking, you see that it is getting brighter and brighter, and then the hallway ends in a beautiful room.

This room is filled with windows, several of which are cracked open just a bit, allowing a nice, cool, refreshing breeze to flow through the room. Sunlight is streaming in through the windows. You walk into the room and there is a big, soft, fluffy couch up against the wall. You decide to sit and then lie down on the couch. Your body is completely supported by the couch, and there is a large, fluffy pillow under your head, and another one under your knees, taking away any tension from your neck and shoulders and back and feet.

As you lie there, you feel the sunlight on your body, covering you from head to toe, warming you, and you feel the cool breeze flowing over you. The combination of the warm sun and the cool breeze makes you feel even more relaxed, and you begin to fall into a deep state of relaxation. You remind yourself this is your time for relaxation. You have nowhere to go and nothing to do. Any thoughts that come into your mind simply flow in and flow out. You don't need to hold onto any thoughts—just let them flow by.

Just outside this room, there are some orange and grapefruit trees. This is a very safe, very relaxing place. Just past the trees is a beach. You begin to think about this beach, and the ocean. You imagine yourself standing at the shoreline, and can feel the wet sand as it goes in between your toes. You look out into the crystal clear water and see that there are the most beautiful fish swimming by. You look at the fish; they are all different colors—purple, turquoise, yellow, and black—and then you see a few starfish on the ocean floor. Then some beautiful stingrays swim by. You like to watch as the water changes the shape of their bodies. You are very relaxed as you watch these fish.

Then you focus on the waves, and watch as they come into the shore and then go out back into the ocean. Flowing in and then flowing out and then just flowing along. Nature is very peaceful.

Lying back on the couch, you think more about these waves. In just a moment, you will imagine a wave coming over your body, and as it does, it will soothe and comfort you, and then it will slowly leave your body, taking away any remaining tension and tightness. The wave can be any color—blue, green, purple, or it can be clear. Imagine the wave slowly going over your toes, feet, and ankles. Then it goes up your legs, knees, and thighs. It goes over your hips, hands, arms, and stomach, all the way up to your shoulders, but not over your neck. The wave is warm and comforting. It hangs out for just a minute, relaxing and soothing all of your muscles. Then the wave begins to leave, taking away all remaining tension, going down your stomach, arms, hands, and hips, all the way down past your thighs, knees, legs, and ankles, and then finally leaves your feet and toes. You are now even more relaxed.

Take a moment to enjoy this relaxation, noticing how calm and slow your breathing is. In just a minute, count to 10, and imagine yourself climbing up a set of stairs. With each step, you become more and more alert, but still very relaxed. At the top of the stairs, there will be an arch-way. You will walk through the archway and then you will be back in your own room, taking with you all of the feelings of relaxation.

One, take the first step.
Two, take the second step.
Three, take the third step.
Four, take the fourth step.
Five, take the fifth step.
Six, take the sixth step.
Seven, take the seventh step.
Eight, take the eighth step.
Nine, take the ninth step.
And 10, take the tenth step.

Walk through the archway, and you are back in your room. Remind yourself that you can become this relaxed anytime you'd like, and it will only take 5 minutes!

You can practice relaxing imagery with this scene or with any other relaxing scene. Your parents' book has a few more scenes like this that they'll read to you. Another thing you can do is to use your creativity and come up with your own relaxing scene! It can be anywhere you'd like—it can be a real place (maybe a place you've been) or a made-up one. The only rule is that this place needs to be free of stress and completely relaxing to you.

Mindfulness Meditation

Mindfulness means that you are aware, fully aware, of yourself, and what is happening inside and outside of you. It is when your mind and your body are connected. When you practice mindfulness, you learn how to be present in the moment that you are in. The opposite is when you are doing one thing, but thinking about something else. For example, if you are sitting in class, but thinking about what you will be doing over the weekend, you are not being *mindful* because your focus is not in the place you are in. When you are doing cartwheels or kicking a ball, and all of your attention is on what you are doing, you are being mindful—you are just in the moment you are in.

When you have anxiety or worries, it can cause you to have trouble being in the moment you are in. If you are lying in bed at night worrying about what bad things might happen, your mind is not focused on what it feels like to be in bed or how good it feels for your body to be resting.

Meditation is something that many people, and kids, love to do. It is when you are completely relaxed and you learn how to just be in the place you are *without* thinking. It is like mindfulness, but it goes a bit deeper. When meditating, you are calm in your body and tuning into the sounds and space around you. You are in a place of awareness—just being aware of your body and what it's like to "be." It sounds like something that is learned, but really it's the most natural thing in the world because when you were born, you did not think at first. You would just see things around you and be in the moment you were in. So, "learning" how to meditate really is just knowing how to be like you were before you were thinking all the time, and before you had anxiety!

Your parent will practice this with you and will read you a script that guides you through a practice. You may even listen to a recording on mindfulness or mindfulness meditation. Learning how to do this is really wonderful because it will not only help you feel calmer and better, it will also help you be able to "sit with" the discomfort and bad feelings that come up when you are anxious. So, it will actually help you be better able to do the steps on your ladder.

Yoga

Do you know anyone who does yoga? Have you ever tried it? Yoga is very relaxing and helps your body be more flexible. It also teaches you how to be in touch with your body and be in the moment you are in. When someone is anxious, he is stuck in his mind. Yoga teaches you how to be more in your body.

The following are three popular poses that are easy to do:

1. Standing Mountain Pose:
   Stand with your feet hip-width apart and your arms down by your sides. Stand up nice and tall and very straight with your shoulders back. Try to get your chest to lift up, as if someone is pulling your chest up with a string that is attached to it.
   Now turn your palms facing out, away from you. Slowly raise your arms, keeping your elbows straight if you can. Once your arms are all the way up, your

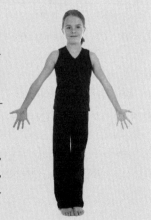

hands will be facing one another, and your fingers will be reaching up toward the sky. Stretch up and reach up as high as you can, while keeping your feet planted firmly into the floor. Try to encourage your upper spine to move into your body and your shoulder blades to move closer together.

Continue to reach up with your fingertips, and push your feet down into the floor, as if your feet were the roots of a tree (your leg muscles should become tight as you do this). Your upper body is stretching up while your lower body is pushing down. As you do this, feel confident about yourself and feel your body opening and lengthening as you stretch and stretch.

2. Downward–Facing Dog Pose:
   Lie facedown on the floor, bend your elbows, and put your hands down on the floor next to your armpits (or chest).

   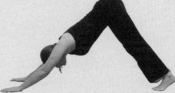

   a. Now get up on all fours (on your hands and knees) and spread your fingers apart, but keep your hands with open palms on the floor.
   b. Now lift up onto your feet, standing mainly on your toes, lifting your hips up, and keeping your hands on the floor. Your hands should be shoulder–width apart.
   c. Continue to lift your hips up and stretch your back. Continue to spread your fingers apart and push your hands against the floor to encourage more lengthening in your spine and more lift in your hips. Hips up, hips up. Feel the stretch.
   d. Very good! Now gently come back down onto all fours, lie back down on your stomach, and relax.

3. Child's Pose:
   Lie facedown on the floor, and touch your big toes together while sitting on the heels of your feet.

   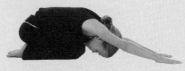

   a. Now spread your knees apart so your knees go out toward the side.

b. Lay your chest on the floor and let your belly sink down toward the floor as well. Your thighs and knees should be out to the side.

c. Stretch your arms and fingers out in front of you with your arms lifting up a few inches above the floor and your fingertips touching the floor. As you do this, try to get your upper back and upper spine to come into your body. Feel the stretch.

d. Now bring your arms down by your sides, with your hands (palms facing up) resting on the floor alongside or below your feet. Just let your entire body relax and rest. Let go of any tension in your body.

Stress Management

One last thing to keep in mind, because it is part of learning how to deal with anxiety, is stress management. The last part of this chapter is about how to manage or deal with stress. There are a few things that everyone should do to lower their stress beaker. What is a beaker, you ask? Well, let me explain.

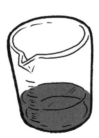

A beaker is a measure of how much stress you have. Everyone always has a little bit of fluid in their beaker, the everyday kinds of things that may be annoying or stressful—like if you're having broccoli for dinner and you don't really like broccoli, or if you forget to hand in your homework, that kind of thing. Then, other things could happen that will make the level go higher. For example, you may get in trouble at home and lose the privilege of watching TV this week, or your parents have a big fight right in front of you, or you may get a bad grade on a test, or your friends were invited to a party and you weren't, or you have to get a shot and you *really* don't like shots, even more than you don't like broccoli! This is going to make the beaker level go way, way up!

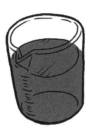

Guess what? Once your beaker is at the top, any little thing— that's right, *any little thing*—can cause it to overflow. When our beakers overflow, we explode, have a meltdown, scream, yell, and cry, whatever. And, guess what else? It's up to *you* to lower your beaker level. It's no one else's job, except yours. Even though your parents, family, and friends can help you feel better, it's really your job to make sure your beaker level doesn't go too high, and certainly doesn't overflow.

Here's what you can do to lower your beaker level:

1. Sleep well (regular bedtime and wake time).
2. Eat well.
3. Exercise.
4. Do yoga.
5. Do relaxation.
6. Express your feelings appropriately.
7. Take a hot bath, and add bubbles if you like.
8. Do 100 jumping jacks or push-ups (after that you'll feel too exhausted to be stressed!).
9. Write in a journal about what is bothering you and what you can do to make it better.
10. Paint a picture or do an art project.

11. Play an instrument.
12. Play with a pet (dog, cat).
13. Distract yourself by reading a book or watching TV or a movie.
14. Call a friend.
15. Play outside.

You are an expert on yourself. You know what other things you can do to make yourself feel better. It is a good idea to think about some other things that make you feel relaxed, such as swinging on a swing, doing yoga, swimming or playing sports, or going outside and taking pictures with a camera. You can write some of your ideas here:

_____

_____

_____

_____

_____

_____

_____

_____

Also remember that, if you tend to worry about schoolwork and getting everything done on time, or if you have a very busy schedule, it is very important to keep up with your school demands because getting behind makes most kids feel stressed out. I also recommend that you have one day each week that you don't do ANY schoolwork, because everyone needs a break and a day to just relax and have fun. You need down-time to be creative. It also feels good to spend time with friends, and this can help you relax, too.

Chapter 3 EXERCISE

Practice Relaxation

Your exercise this week includes:
1. A topic question for you and your parent to talk about.
2. Making a calm breathing note card.
3. Practicing your relaxation 5 days this week.

Try not to think of practicing the relaxation as a chore, but as something that feels very good that you can look forward to doing. Knowing how to relax is one of the most important tools you will use when we get to the "facing your fears" part. Your parent will help you by practicing with you over the week.

Discussion Topic

Talk to your parents about what makes them feel relaxed—what they do to calm down and manage stress. Tell them what makes you feel relaxed and what you think can help you calm down. Your parents might want to know what they can do to help you feel less stressed.

Calm Breathing Note Card

Use one note card to write down how to do calm breathing. Make your note card look like this one:

Calm Breathing

In → nose → count of 4
Hold → count of 4
Out → mouth → count of 4

Then on the back, make yours look like this:

> **Calm Breathing**
>
> Breathe in and out through only one nostril. Hold your other nostril closed and close your mouth.
> Count of 10 in and count of 10 out.

Practice Relaxation

Check off the days that you practiced and what type of relaxation you did in the chart below.

Day of the Week	Calm Breathing	Progressive Muscle Relaxation (PMR)	Relaxing Imagery	Mindfulness Meditation	Yoga
Monday					
Tuesday					
Wednesday					
Thursday					
Friday					
Saturday					
Sunday					

Try to do at least one technique a day and to try each technique at least once this week. If you choose to listen to an app or CD track, check which type of strategy was used.

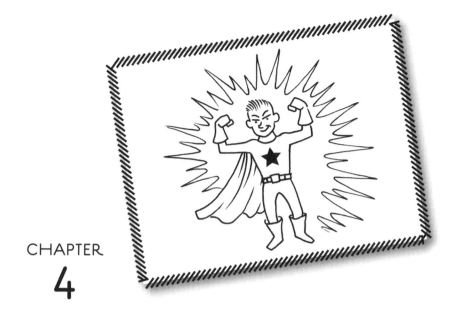

4

Conquer Your Worries

IN this chapter, you will learn how to get rid of your worries. Worries are thoughts (this chapter and the next one are about the thoughts part of anxiety). You will learn that most worrying is a waste of time (although just knowing this is not enough to get rid of them).

There are several ways to conquer worry:
- ▶ understanding the two types of worry,
- ▶ asking yourself two things,
- ▶ positive self-talk,
- ▶ talking back to the anxiety,
- ▶ challenging anticipatory anxiety,
- ▶ schedule "worry time,"

- ▶ worry tapes, and
- ▶ uncertainty training.

Understanding the Two Types of Worry: Useful and Useless Worry

Useful worry is worry that helps you get something done, without causing any of the body signs of anxiety. This type of worry is productive, because it helps you produce something you want to get done. For example, when you have a big assignment in school that you really want to do well on, you spend a good amount of time working on it and worry about how good it will be. This worry is helpful because it helps motivate you to get your work done.

Useless worry is worry that prevents you from getting things done, and causes you to have body signs like tight muscles and an upset stomach. This type of worry is unproductive, because it stops you from doing something. For example, you decide not to go to a sleepover party with your friends because you are worried about being away from your mom or dad.

The most important thing that you should know about useless worry is that its goal is to make you scared and upset when there is no reason to feel this way. Useless worry is "just the anxiety talking." By facing your fears, you are going to get rid of your anxiety! You will be able to do this because when you face your fears, you will see that there was nothing to worry about in the first place.

Worrying makes you feel a fake sense of control. It becomes a habit, which means you get used to thinking these worries. I know that when you look back at all of the things you have worried about, you will find that most of them never happened.

Asking Yourself Two Things

When you are worried, ask yourself the following two questions:
1. What is the worst thing that could happen?
2. Could I handle it?

When answering the first question, try to come up a few different possibilities. Think about what could happen and come up with a list in your head. For example, say you are worried about a test tomorrow and how you will do on it. The answer to the first question might be: I would fail the test and get a lower grade in the class, and if this happened, my parents would be upset about my report card and I might get in trouble. Usually we think about what might happen and it is not really possible. For example, some kids in middle school worry that if they don't do well on one test they won't get into college, and this worry is not possible. One test will not prevent you from getting into college, plus colleges don't look at middle school report cards! Now let's say that you are worried about germs. You might think that the worst thing that could happen from touching doorknobs is that you will get germs on you, but if you thought that you would get sick and die, that would not be possible. People cannot get sick and die from touching doorknobs (if so, everyone would die because we all touch doorknobs to open doors)! So, when you think of the "worst thing that could happen," only list things that could really happen. Mom or Dad or another adult can help you decide what could really happen if you are not sure.

Guess what the answer to the second question is. It starts with Y.

"Yes!" The answer is *always* "yes," because you can handle anything. There is nothing in life that you cannot handle. You are resilient!

Positive Self-Talk

Self-talk is what you say to yourself (this is part of your thoughts, so it's likely that you probably don't talk to yourself out loud). When you are feeling anxious, your thoughts are filled with worries and negative self-talk. Here are some examples of negative self-talk:

"I can't do it."

"I can't handle this."

"I won't be OK."

"It's going to be terrible"

"I need to be with Mom or Dad to feel safe."

"This is too scary."

"I'm too nervous to do this."

When you tell yourself these kinds of things, you will become even more nervous and scared. However, if you use positive self-talk, you will be able to get through a scary situation and you will feel less nervous and scared. Here are some examples of positive self-talk:

"I must face my fears to overcome them. I can do it!"

"I can handle this. I am nervous, but I am OK."

"I am scared, but I am safe."

"I am OK. Everything will work out."

"I can handle whatever comes my way."

"I can change the way I think to change the way I feel."

"It is my choice to be calm or be nervous. I am choosing to be calm. Let me start by calming my breath."

"Anxiety is not an accurate predictor of what's to come. Anxiety is just an unpleasant feeling."

"It's just the anxiety talking. I don't have to listen to it."

"What would someone without anxiety think in this situation? What would they do?"

"What would someone without OCD think in this situation? What would they do?"

"What would someone who is completely confident do in this situation?"

Many kids will use positive self-talk, even though they don't necessarily believe what they are telling themselves at first. But with practice, you will see that these statements are true! The more you practice this kind of self-talk, the more you will feel like you can handle situations that make you feel anxious.

Talking Back to the Anxiety

Part of self-talk is learning how to "talk back" to the anxiety. Although it is not good behavior to talk back to your parents, teachers, or other adults, it is very good of you to talk back to the anxiety. It is important to realize that you and the anxiety are not the same. The anxiety is a separate thing, even though it often feels like it is part of you. Think of the anxiety as external or outside of you—something separate. And, when you have scary thoughts or useless worry, say to yourself, "It is just the anxiety talking" and remind yourself that you don't need to listen to it. If you listen to it, the anxiety will win and get stronger, but if you don't listen to it, you will win and get stronger!

Challenging Anticipatory Anxiety

Anticipatory anxiety is when you feel nervous or scared about something before it happens. Anticipating something means that you are waiting for it to happen. For example, let's say that going on class field trips makes you anxious. When you hear that you are going on one tomorrow, you may be nervous and worried all day and all night, *before* the field trip occurs. In other words, you are worrying about something before it happens—and this is anticipa-tory anxiety. Let's say that you get very nervous when your parents go out of town, and they tell you that they are going away for the weekend. As soon as you learn about their plans, you may begin to feel very anxious and scared, even though they haven't left yet! This is called anticipatory anxiety because you are waiting for (or "anticipating") something to happen that you feel is going to be scary.

Most of the worrying you do is about something that is *going* to happen, not something that already has happened. So, most of your worrying is really anticipatory anxiety. If you are going to see the doctor, you may worry about getting a shot. You may cry, scream, or have a meltdown, because you are so worried about the possibility of getting a shot. This is anticipatory anxiety. Once you get to the doctor's office, you may be told that you don't need any shots, or you may be told that you do need one. Let's say that you do get the shot—most kids realize that even though they don't like them, shots are not as bad as they thought they would be.

Now that you understand what anticipatory anxiety is, let me tell you what you can do to deal with it. There are three steps to dealing or coping with anticipatory anxiety:

1. Label your worries and scary feelings as "anticipatory anxi-ety." Say to yourself, "It is just anticipatory anxiety, and anxiety is not a good predictor of what's to come."

2. Replace these thoughts with healthier, more balanced thoughts. Use positive self-talk to reassure yourself that you will be OK and that you can handle what comes your way (e.g., "I will be OK and I can handle what comes my way").

3. Remind yourself to "be proactive." Proactive people do not allow anxiety to make decisions for them or influence their behavior (although reactive people do).

Schedule "Worry Time"

Another thing you can do to conquer worry is to schedule *worry time*. This means you set a time each day that you will worry on purpose. You should schedule between 10–20 minutes for worry time, and you can do it once or twice a day. If you worry a lot, you will want to set up two times—maybe once after school and then once after dinner.

Worry time teaches you to "get your worries out" in a planned way, and you learn that you can hold off on worrying until it's time for worry time. Also, many kids figure out that their worries are the same day after day, and the worries start to seem useless and even sort of boring.

When you are doing worry time, it is very important that you use the whole time and not stop before it's over. Even if you run out of things to worry about, try to keep thinking of new things, and if you can't think of anything else, then just stay where you are until the time is up. Sometimes you will remember other worries, but sometimes you might end up just sitting there until the worry time ends.

There are a few different ways to worry during worry time. You can say your worries out loud to a parent, write them down, or type them up in list form. Another option is to make a worry tape, which is really the best technique to use for conquering your worries or anxious thoughts that keep coming up over and over in your head.

Worry Tapes

When making a worry tape, you can use a digital recorder or an easier option if you have a smartphone is to use the voice recorder option (for iPhones, it's under Utilities: Voice Memos). Many kids first type out a script of their worries that they read from: They list their worries and then read from the list while recording them. Other kids just talk about their worries and record them without a script. Either way, it is very important to record the worries exactly how they sound in your head. For example, instead of recording "Sometimes I worry that a dog will bite me," you would say, "What if that dog bites me?" because that is how worries really sound when you have them.

Once the recording is at least one minute long, you can start to listen to it. The goal is to listen to it over and over until the worries start to sound boring. At first, you will most likely feel anxious or more worried from listening, but it will get easier. When you listen over and over, your anxiety will go away and the thoughts won't seem alarming anymore. If you get anxious in the beginning, you want to practice "sitting with" the uncomfortable feelings and tolerate the bad feelings. It's important to do this so you can eventually become used to hearing the recording. When listening, if you have more worries come up, just write them down and make another recording.

The goal is to listen to the worry recording for 10–20 minutes every day, for at least 2 weeks; most kids need to listen to it for 4 weeks to become completely bored by the thoughts. Try to keep your focus on the recording, and if you get distracted, then you should pause it until you can refocus. It only works if you are actually hearing the worries!

When Billy made a worry loop, he spoke into the recorder and said, "What if I can't get my work done? I'm worried that I will have to stay in for recess. What if Mom doesn't let me stay home tomorrow and I have to take the test?" Billy made his worries sound just like they sounded when he thinks his worries. Once you record your worries, you can listen to the recording over and over during each worry time. Many kids end up adding onto the tape or digital recording as they think of more worries. The worry recording helps make the worries less powerful, and by listening to it over and over, you will be able to get rid of your worries!

Uncertainty Training

Anxiety and worries are usually about what *might* happen, not what actually will happen. So, when you learn how to be OK with not knowing for sure what might happen, then you will be better at handling your worries. Uncertainty training is when you practice being OK with not knowing for sure what will happen. Uncertainty training will teach you how to *tolerate* uncertainty.

To do uncertainty training, you can make a second loop recording, but this time instead of just listing the worries and the "what if . . ." thoughts, you would repeat: "It is always possible that . . ." whatever you are afraid of will happen. So, if you are afraid of dogs, you would say: "It is always possible that the dog will jump on me. It is always possible that a dog will bite me. It is always possible I'll be really scared of a dog and cry." When you say your worries this way, not only are you getting use to the thoughts about what might happen, you are becoming more comfortable with the idea of **not knowing** what will happen.

After you make an uncertainty training recording, you can listen to this right after your worry tape recording. Most kids don't like doing these recordings or listening to them, but they realize how useful they are at getting rid of the worries. This is another way to make the worries lose their power over you and your life.

EXERCISE

Chapter 4 EXERCISE

Self-Talk Note Cards and Worry Tapes

Your exercise this week includes:

1. Making 8–10 self-talk note cards.
2. Making a list: "When the anxiety talks, it says . . ."
3. Make a recording (either worry tape or uncertainty training, or both).
4. Keep practicing your relaxation (try to do it at least three times this week).

Self-Talk Note Cards

When making your note cards, you can use different colored index cards and you can add stickers to the note cards if you'd like. You can write them or have your parent write them—it's your choice. You will make seven note cards like the ones on the next page, and also make three to five cards of your own (you can make more if you'd like, but try to make at least three extra cards). The ones that you make on your own should be specific to you; they should be things that you can say to yourself that will help with your own specific worries and anxieties. Your parent will help you with what to write.

Seven note cards to make (make yours look just like these) are on the next page.

It's the Anxiety Talking

Remember James, the boy who was afraid of snakes? Well, when his anxiety was talking, it said things like:

"Snakes are scary and they bite."

"Don't go near the bushes, because a snake could be in there."

"That rustling sound was a snake."

"You can't go near snakes—they are the worst!"

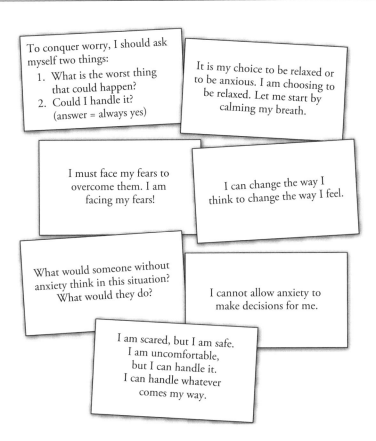

To conquer worry, I should ask myself two things:
1. What is the worst thing that could happen?
2. Could I handle it?
   (answer = always yes)

It is my choice to be relaxed or to be anxious. I am choosing to be relaxed. Let me start by calming my breath.

I must face my fears to overcome them. I am facing my fears!

I can change the way I think to change the way I feel.

What would someone without anxiety think in this situation? What would they do?

I cannot allow anxiety to make decisions for me.

I am scared, but I am safe.
I am uncomfortable,
but I can handle it.
I can handle whatever
comes my way.

James had to learn how to talk back to his anxiety, and he did this by knowing when his anxiety was talking to him and choosing not to listen to it! He told himself that the anxiety was wrong, then he told himself different things to help himself be able to face his fears. For example, he told himself that the rustling sound was most likely a squirrel or a bird. He reminded himself that most snakes don't bite humans. This is how he was able to face his fears and overcome his fear of snakes.

EXERCISE

In the space below, write in some of the things that the anxiety says when you are feeling scared or anxious:

"When my anxiety talks, it says . . ."

_____

_____

_____

_____

Make a Recording

Write down all of your worries, just as they sound in your head. You can use what you wrote above for "When my anxiety talks, it says . . . ". Then record your worries on a phone or digital recorder (have your parent help you with the set up). When doing the recording, remember to make it sound exactly as it sounds in your head. For example, let's say you are afraid of a dog jumping on you, then you would record the thought as it sounds when you think it: "What if that dog jumps on me?" (you wouldn't say "Sometimes I worry that a dog will jump on me"). We want it to sound just like it sounds in your head, so the recording should be in your voice.

You can do a worry tape or an uncertainty training recording ("It is always possible that a dog will jump on me"), or both. It is best to do both and then listen to both recordings. Remember that it gets worse before it gets easier, and that while many people don't like to hear the worries on a recording, when you listen to it over and over for 10–20 minutes a day for 2–4 weeks, your worries will become boring to you. Doing this works 100% of the time!

_____

_____

_____

Practice Relaxation

Use the chart in the previous chapter to check off the days that you practiced and what type of relaxation you did.

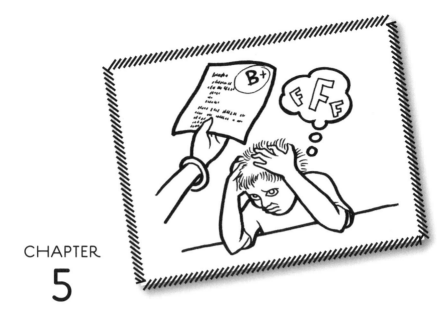

5

Changing Your Thoughts

I N this chapter, you will learn about the different types of anxious thinking. You also will learn how to change your anxious thoughts and beliefs and change your relationship with your thoughts (as a reminder, this chapter also is about the thoughts part of anxiety).

Let's start by understanding the connection between your thoughts and feelings. The way you think about a situation affects how you will feel about it, and how you behave. For example, if you think that playing with your neighbor's dog is a lot of fun, you will feel excited about it. But, if you think that playing with your neighbor's dog is scary and frightening, you will feel nervous about it and will avoid playing with the dog.

Situation →	Thoughts →	Feelings →	Actions
You are in front of your house and your neighbor is outside with her dog.	I really like dogs and can't wait to play with Charlie. He's so cute!	Excited Happy Eager	Go outside and pet Charlie.

Situation →	Thoughts →	Feelings →	Actions
You are in front of your house and your neighbor is outside with her dog.	Dogs are so scary! I hope he doesn't come near me. If he comes toward me, I'll run inside!	Anxious Nervous Scared	Stay inside or run away from Charlie if he comes near you.

Situation →	Thoughts →	Feelings →	Actions
You are called on in class by the teacher to answer a question.	I feel comfortable being called on. I like to share my thoughts. Maybe the teacher will like my answer.	Relaxed Calm Enthusiastic	Comfortably and naturally share your ideas.

Situation →	Thoughts →	Feelings →	Actions
You are called on in class by the teacher to answer a question.	I can't stand talking in front of the class. What if I say the wrong answer and everyone laughs and thinks I'm dumb?	Anxious Nervous Scared	Quietly say, "I don't know," or limit what you say.

Situation →	Thoughts →	Feelings →	Actions
You have a big science test tomorrow and you have been studying for 3 days.	I am prepared and will probably do well because I have been studying a lot.	Calm Self-Assured Organized	Take the test, focusing on trying your best.

Situation →	Thoughts →	Feelings →	Actions
You have a big science test tomorrow and you have been studying for 3 days.	What if I fail? What if I forget everything I know? I will be in big trouble if I fail. The test is going to be impossible!	Anxious Nervous Scared	Have trouble sleeping the night before and ask your parents for reassurance.

The examples above show that if something makes you feel anxious, it has to do with the way you are thinking about it. This also means that you can *change the way you think to change the way you feel*! This is a very important step in overcoming your worry and anxiety. You can do this, and the more you practice, the better you will become.

Can you imagine what would happen if the child in the above example were to change his thoughts and begin thinking like a nonanxious person? So, once the thoughts about failing the science test come up (and he thinks about how hard it will be and how he will get in big trouble if he fails), he would *change* these thoughts to thoughts like "I am prepared. I will probably do well because I have been studying a lot." In the beginning, he may not believe what he is telling himself; however, as he keeps practicing this type of thinking, it eventually will become natural and automatic.

Part of changing your thoughts involves learning the type of thinking mistakes you are making that are causing you to feel anxious and nervous. It is also important to know that your thoughts don't have any power, unless you give them power.

Types of Thinking Mistakes

All humans make thinking mistakes, also called thinking errors—this includes all kids and all adults. Thinking errors are thoughts that you have automatically that cause you to feel bad and anxious. Thinking errors are thoughts that are wrong or incorrect;

they are rooted in anxiety. Don't feel bad for making thinking mistakes—remember, all kids and all adults make them. Let me give you a personal example:

Years ago, I was visiting an island called Barbados and heard that there were really cool sea turtles in the ocean. The only thing was that you needed to take a speedboat to get to see them. Well, when the motorboat came up to the ocean shore to pick us up, I suddenly felt a rush of anxiety and fear and worry come over me. My heart started pounding, my stomach and knees felt weak, and I couldn't stop thinking about how scary it would feel going so fast on this boat—speeding along on the ocean. And I kept thinking that the boat was going so far from shore and what if it broke down and we got stuck out there? I really felt too afraid to go. I told my husband, Brian, that I was so nervous that I wasn't sure I could go and that I might not go and he replied, "Well, you need to face your fears, just like the kids you work with," then he jumped onto the boat! I decided to take his (really my) advice and got on the boat too. The next thing I knew, we were speeding along on the ocean going very fast and the funny thing was, I had no anxiety at all! Not even the tiniest amount of fear. I probably couldn't have felt afraid if I tried. I was totally calm and relaxed and loved every minute of the boat ride. I loved the feeling of the ocean air against my face, the feeling of being on a boat, traveling on water, and looking at the beautiful island as we rode by. More than all of this, swimming with the sea turtles was one of the greatest times of my life! The sea turtles were huge and so interesting to watch as they swam in their ocean. It was a magical time and it would never have happened if I didn't face my fears.

As you can see, the thoughts I had about going on the boat and my body's feelings of anxiety were not good predictors of what being on the boat would be like. My thoughts were not correct; they were wrong—they were thinking mistakes. I was making two types of thinking errors: "probability overestimations" and "catastrophizing." Sometimes one thought will actually include more than one thinking mistake.

Let me tell you about 10 different types of thinking errors and give you examples of each. Most kids tend to make several of these thinking errors. When reading about them, try to think about which ones you make:

1. **Catastrophizing:** Visualizing disaster; thinking that the worst thing is going to happen and feeling like you wouldn't be able to handle it; asking "What if . . . "
   a. *Example:* What if I am scared on the motorboat and won't be able to calm down?
   b. *Example:* You parents are going out for dinner without you and you think that something bad will happen to them or to you. What if they get hurt?

2. **All-or-Nothing:** Also known as black-and-white thinking, dichotomous thinking, and polarized thinking; thinking in extremes—things are either perfect or a failure; there is no middle ground—it's either one extreme or another; thinking in an inflexible way.
   a. *Example:* If I don't get an A on this test, I will fail the whole class and have a terrible report card.
   b. *Example:* You and your family planned on having pizza for dinner, but your mom brings home Chinese food instead. You are so upset and tell your mom, "The whole day is ruined now! I didn't want Chinese!"

3. **Filtering:** Focusing on the negative parts of a situation while ignoring the positive parts; catching all of the bad

parts and forgetting about the good parts; disqualifying the positive.

a. *Example:* You go to a birthday party and have a great time until the end when another kid says something mean to you. Your dad picks you up and asks how the party was and you tell him, "It was terrible. I had the worst time!"

b. *Example:* You get your report card and make all A's and B's but got a C in history. You feel so upset and only think about your history grade; you ignore all the other good grades that you earned.

4. **Magnifying:** Making something seem bigger and worse than it really is; turning up the volume on anything bad, making it worse.

a. *Example:* Your dad reminds you that you have a check-up at the doctor's tomorrow after school. You begin to cry and you tell him that this is the worst news you have ever heard!

b. *Example:* A bug lands on your shirt and you scream at the top of your lungs and run around trying to get it off.

5. **Shoulds:** Rules that you have about how things should be; using the words "should," "must," and "ought to" to show how things should be.

a. *Example:* You make a mistake and forget to hand in an assignment. When you hand it in the next day, your teacher marks it down to a B because it is late. You feel so upset with yourself and think, "I shouldn't make mistakes like this. That was so stupid of me."

b. *Example:* A friend comes over to play and you think that she should play with whatever games you pick, because you're playing at your house. You pick out Monopoly but she tells you that she doesn't want to play Monopoly and would rather play Clue. You become very upset with her because you believe that she should follow your rules.

6. **Mind Reading:** Thinking you know what others are thinking, particularly what they are thinking about you; usually you will think that others are thinking negatively about you.
   a. *Example:* When you are answering a question in class, you think that other kids are thinking that you are stupid and don't know what you are talking about.
   b. *Example:* When your baseball coach gives you a pointer, you think that he thinks you are the worst player on the team.

7. **Overgeneralization:** Taking a single incident and thinking that it will always be this way; something happens once and you think it will always happen this way.
   a. *Example:* You give a presentation on your book report and you feel very nervous throughout the presentation. Afterward, you tell yourself that anytime you give a presentation you are going to feel very nervous.
   b. *Example:* You go to an awards ceremony at school, but don't get any awards. When leaving, you tell your parents that you're never going to an awards ceremony again because you won't get an award anyway!

8. **Personalization:** Taking something personally; making it about you when it has nothing to do with you.
   a. *Example:* You walk by two girls in the lunchroom and they are whispering, so you think that they are whispering about you.
   b. *Example:* You didn't receive an invitation to your friend's birthday party, so you think that he must be mad at you and doesn't want to be your friend anymore.

9. **Selective Attention:** Paying attention to things that confirm your beliefs about something; ignoring evidence that goes against what you believe about a particular situation.
   a. *Example:* You think that other kids don't like you and then you remember the time you were teased at recess and when your neighbor told you she didn't want to play with you anymore. You don't think about the kids who do like you or about all of the fun you have with your friends from soccer after school.
   b. *Example:* Your brother gets a new computer and this makes you think about how your mom and dad don't get you anything, and how your computer is 2 years old. You don't think about how you recently got a new bed and that when you got your computer 2 years ago, your brother did not get one.

10. **Probability Overestimation:** Overestimating the likelihood that something bad will happen.
    a. *Example:* You think that your presentation is going to be terrible and that you will be panicked the whole time.
    b. *Example:* You are about to get on a motorboat and you think that you will be scared and anxious during the whole ride (does this sound familiar?).

Replacing Your Anxious Thoughts

After you have identified what your anxious thoughts are, the next step is to change them. You can do this by replacing your thoughts with balanced, neutral thoughts. For example, instead of thinking that others are thinking bad things about you, you can think that most likely they are not having bad thoughts about you. Instead of thinking about something bad happening to your parents, you can think about how they go out to dinner all of the time and are always safe. Instead of thinking that the whole day is ruined because your mom brought home Chinese food and not pizza, you can think about the day more realistically and how the rest of the day can be great (maybe not the food part, but the rest of it).

To replace your thoughts, you want to consider the facts and ask yourself, "What proof do I have that this thought is correct?" For example, what proof do you have that your mind reading is correct? How do you know that the other kids think you are stupid when you are answering a question in class? How do you know how you will feel once you are speeding along the water on a motorboat? What proof do you have that your presentation will be a disaster? Even if you have given not-so-great presentations in the past, how do you know that this particular presentation won't go well? The *fact* is that you don't have any proof about what will happen in the future, because it hasn't happened yet! Remember, your worries are part of anticipatory anxiety; they are about future events that haven't occurred yet.

Challenge your anxious thoughts by asking yourself, "What would someone who is not anxious in this situation think right now?" or "What would someone who is completely secure in this situation think right now?"

Changing Your Relationship With Your Anxious Thoughts

Another way of getting rid of your anxious thoughts it to actually change your relationship with them. That may sounds a little funny because we usually don't go around thinking about the relationship we have with our thoughts, but it's just about seeing your thoughts differently. Thoughts don't have any power on their own—they are just thoughts. They only have power if we give them power, which means we can also take their power over us away.

"Detached mindfulness" is a technique that teaches you how to become aware (mindful) of and separate (detached) from your anxious thoughts by learning how to become an observer of them. When you become an observer of your thoughts, you see yourself having the anxious thoughts and are better able to view them as "just thoughts." You go from just listening to your thoughts to seeing yourself having the thoughts.

Once you see the anxious thoughts for what they are, you will be able to classify them as part of the anxiety, rather than thoughts that count. Whether a thought is true or not, it's just a thought and nothing else. In detached mindfulness, you don't try to change the thought; you just try to change how you experience the thought. The goal is for you to no longer listen to what the thought is saying—rather you just see the thought as a part of the anxiety. This way, it allows you to dismiss the anxious thoughts.

To help you learn detached mindfulness, take 10 sheets or paper and write down 10 different thoughts. Try to come up with seven neutral/common thoughts, two anxiety thoughts, and one untrue thought. Then, read the 10 thoughts three times in a row, quickly. Once you read the thoughts three times in a row, say aloud: "I can see these are just thoughts. Whether they are true or not, neutral or scary, they are just thoughts. Thoughts do not have any power unless I give them power." It is best to practice this 1–2 times a day for a few weeks.

Here are examples of 10 thoughts:

"I love pepperoni pizza from Ledo's. Maybe I'll have it this weekend." (N)
"The fall is my favorite season—the leaves are so amazing." (N)
"I have a big test next week and will have to study a lot for it." (N)
"What if someone breaks in and kills us all?" (A)
"Over winter break we are going to Florida. I can't wait." (N)

"I will probably join the animal rights club that's starting soon." (N)

"I'm wearing neon green socks." (U)

"My favorite book is the Harry Potter series." (N)

"What if there is another terrorist attack?" (A)

"I love my brother. We have the best time playing together." (N)

(N = neutral, A = anxiety-provoking, U = untrue)

The most brilliant feedback I received from a 13-year-old with OCD who mastered this technique was when he told me, "I think I got it. Now, when the terrible thoughts come up, I see them as if they are being typed out on a screen in front of me; I cannot really read them or know them, but I see it as just the OCD and it doesn't bother me anymore." With practice, you can also learn to become an observer of your anxious thoughts and therefore, not be bothered by them.

EXERCISE

Chapter 5 EXERCISE

Identify and Replace Thinking Errors

Your exercise this week includes:

1. Listing two of your anxiety situations from your ladder and the anxious thoughts you have about these situations.

2. Labeling your thinking mistakes if there are any.

3. Changing your thoughts by creating "replacement thoughts," using the tool on the next few pages to write down your old and new thoughts. Remember: Replacement thoughts are balanced and neutral thoughts that do not cause anxiety. (*Hint*: You will know that you came up with a good replacement thought when the thought makes you feel calmer and more prepared to cope with the scary situation.)

4. Make 10 cards for detached mindfulness. Write down 10 different thoughts (seven of which are typical, neutral thoughts; two of which are anxious thoughts; and one untrue thought). Mix them up and read them 3 times in a row quickly each day. After reading them, each time say aloud: "I can see these are just thoughts. Whether they are true or not, neutral or scary, they are just thoughts. Thoughts do not have any power unless I give them power." Do this for 2–3 weeks (it shouldn't take more than 3 minutes a day).

Situation →	Thoughts →	Thinking Error(s)

Replacement Thoughts:

EXERCISE

Situation →	Thoughts →	Thinking Error(s)

Replacement Thoughts:

Situation →	Thoughts →	Thinking Error(s)

Replacement Thoughts:

EXERCISE

Situation →	Thoughts →	Thinking Error(s)

Replacement Thoughts:

Write your 10 thoughts for Detached Mindfulness practice here:

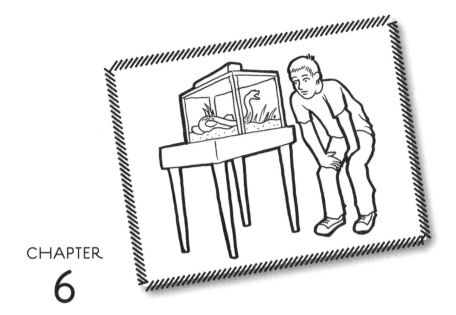

CHAPTER

6

Changing Your Behaviors

Facing Your Fears

I N this chapter, we will focus on preparing you to face your fears! So, this chapter is about the behavior part of anxiety. You have already learned about the body and thoughts parts and are now ready for this last part: behavior.

The last chapter showed you that your thoughts impact your feelings and actions. It also is true that your feelings impact your behavior. If you *feel* scared of something, you probably are going to try to avoid it—and avoidance is a behavior. There are other behaviors that kids often do when they are feeling scared or anxious. These include:

▶   reassurance seeking (asking your mom or dad or someone else to tell you that you're OK);

- ► asking a lot of questions;
- ► overplanning activities;
- ► repeating information or previously answered questions;
- ► clinging (staying near your parent or another adult);
- ► crying;
- ► picking (nails, hair, feet, lips, or any other part of your body);
- ► fidgeting (moving around a lot or playing with your fingers or hair);
- ► freezing up;
- ► having a tantrum or meltdown;
- ► scanning your environment (looking around for something to make you feel calmer); and
- ► rituals (things you do repeatedly).

As you have learned, avoiding scary situations strengthens your anxiety about the situations. To overcome your anxiety, you cannot do avoidance behavior anymore. Remember: It is you versus your fear. Take a positive attitude and tell yourself that you will win against your fears! As mentioned earlier, you will start facing your fears with the easier and less anxiety-provoking situations and then gradually move up the ladder to harder ones. When you face your fears, you are doing what is called an *exposure*, because you are exposing yourself to the scary situation.

Keep in mind that most kids don't really feel ready to face their fears, they just do the exposures, even if they have to break them down into smaller steps. Your parent should encourage you and might give you a push to do it. Also remember that you are now better prepared to handle facing your fears. You will face your fears by using your coping tools and getting support from your parent. As you face your fears, it also is important to feel good about yourself and compliment yourself. You will reward yourself after facing each fear by putting stickers on your ladder (your parent will do this with you).

A note about getting stars/stickers on your ladder: You can earn two stars for each step on your ladder (each one goes on each side of the ladder for each step). The first star will be earned after you take the step for the first time. You will put the second star on the ladder for that step after you have practiced it enough and it doesn't make you feel anxious or scared anymore. The second star shows that you have overcome your fear for that situation.

I also have some very good news to share with you: Once you are done facing all of your fears, there will be a celebration in your honor. You and your parent(s) are going to have a little party to celebrate you and all of your hard work! You may even get an award or a special treat! You might decide to invite a sibling if you have one or a best friend or grandparent to celebrate you with you and your parent.

OK, so let's start facing your fears by making a **plan for coping**. A plan for coping with the exposures will help you feel prepared to do so. The exercise for this week is going to help you to remember all of the things you can do to manage or cope with your anxiety. It is normal to feel anxiety as you begin to face your fears. But, most kids find that after feeling some anxiety at first, their anxiety goes way down and usually goes away completely. It will be helpful to remind yourself of this fact. The kids I work with always feel great after facing their fears, and usually they find that it was nothing like they expected it to be—in fact, it was much easier. Finding that facing your fears isn't so bad will help motivate you to continue to face your fears that are higher on the ladder in a step-by-step way.

Plan for Coping

A plan for coping will always include using the tools in your "toolbox." The tools are the strategies that you have learned in the previous chapters that help you deal with your anxiety. You will review the tools in your toolbox during the exercise at the end of this chapter. The tools you have include:

- ▶ calm breathing;
- ▶ one-nostril breathing;
- ▶ progressive muscle relaxation;
- ▶ relaxing imagery;
- ▶ asking two important questions;
- ▶ using positive self-talk (read the cards);
- ▶ talking back to the anxiety;
- ▶ dealing with anticipatory anxiety;
- ▶ changing your thoughts (identifying and replacing thinking errors as they come up); and
- ▶ seeing the thoughts as just thoughts and being an observer of the thoughts (detached mindfulness).

Most likely, you won't use *every* tool in your toolbox, just your favorite and most helpful ones. Plus, you may use different tools for different situations. For example, James (the boy who had a snake phobia) used calm breathing as he looked at pictures of snakes in a book, but he used positive self-talk when he stood near a live snake and challenged his catastrophizing thinking.

Sometimes kids are too nervous to use tools to conquer worry and change their thoughts. If this happens, you can use distraction techniques in addition to calm breathing to calm down enough to be able to conquer worries and change your thoughts. Examples of distraction techniques include:

- ▶ Make lists using the ABCs: Go through the alphabet and try to come up with lists alphabetically. For example, girls' names (Aileen, Bonnie, Camryn, Denise, Emily, Frances); cities/states/countries (Alabama, Baltimore, Cuba, Delaware, Ecuador, Florida); jobs (artist, baker, chemist, dentist, engineer, firefighter). It can be any topic and if the alphabetizing is too challenging, you can do the lists without doing them in alphabetical order. This will help distract you from the anxiety-provoking situation.

▶ Focus on something that you can see (for example, a tree, book, your sneakers) and try to think of five or more different parts of it or ways to describe it (for example, What color is it? What shape is it? What does it smell like? What does it sound like? What does it feel like? What could you use it for?).

▶ Pick a color and think of five things that come in that color.

▶ List five favorite books, five favorite songs, or five favorite movies.

▶ Count backward from 100 by 7 (100, 93, 86, 79, . . .) or any other number.

Another part of making a plan for coping during exposures is to decide if you want to break down your exposure into even smaller steps. For instance, when James did his first exposure (talking about snakes) he began by talking about snakes for 1 minute, then did it again the next day for 5 minutes, then did it again on the third day for 10 minutes.

When facing your fears, review what your plan will involve. Think about which tools you will use and which distraction techniques you will rely on if you have a hard time focusing on using your tools.

When it comes time for you to do an exposure, rate how anxious or scared you were on a scale from 0 to 10. We can think of this scale as a FEAR-mometer, sort of like a thermometer that measures temperature, but this measures fear.

    0 = no fear at all/completely relaxed like in a deep sleep

    5 = nervous and scared but not too terrible

  10 = extremely afraid, totally anxious, and panicked

Chapter 6 EXERCISE

Facing Your Fears

Your exercise this week includes:

1. Drawing a picture of a toolbox and writing the different "tools" in it on your own paper (remember the tools are the different strategies you can use to manage your anxiety; they are all listed earlier in this chapter).

2. Taking the first step of your ladder (do your first exposure).

   a. Remember to put stickers on your ladder after you have practiced your first step several times.

   b. Remember to note what your anxiety level was on the FEAR-mometer.

Make your picture of the toolbox look something like this one:

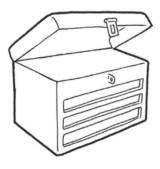

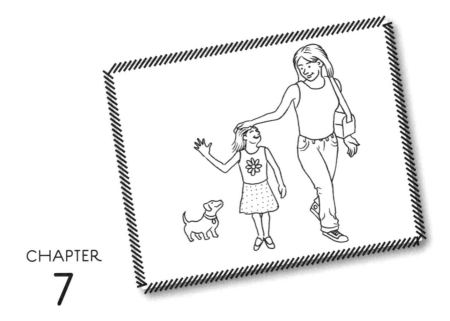

CHAPTER

7

Keep Facing Your Fears and Build Confidence

THIS is another short chapter that also is on behavior. If you are reading this chapter, it most likely means that you have faced your first fear, so let me say "Congratulations!" This was a big step and you should feel very proud of yourself for getting this far. I am certainly proud of you!

As you can probably guess, the exercise at the end of this chapter is going to be taking the rest of the steps on your ladder, one at a time. Once you finish taking all of the steps on your ladder, you can go onto the next chapter (which is the last chapter) and celebrate.

Remember that although it is going to be hard to do many of the steps on your ladder, you will feel so much better once you do them and you will be free to live your life without anxiety controlling it. You also will feel better about yourself. Before we talk more about the behavior part, let's talk a little about the idea of feeling proud of yourself.

Self-esteem refers to how you feel about yourself; it can be positive or negative. Kids with good self-esteem mostly feel good about who they are and feel proud of their accomplishments. They know that while it feels good for others to think positively about them, it has to come from the inside, too.

The way you think has a lot to do with your self-esteem. For example, kids who believe that if they work hard and stick with a challenging task, then they will learn more or get better at doing it end up feeling better about themselves in the end. The opposite would be thinking that it doesn't matter how hard you try, you won't get better at it. Kids who know that they can do something to change a difficult situation also have more confidence. The opposite would be feeling that there is nothing you can do. You can *always* do something to change an unpleasant situation, even if it's just changing how you feel about it.

Most kids have some trouble with friends at some point when growing up. When other kids are mean or tease you, you have to be "assertive" and stick up for yourself. Ignoring doesn't work and actually lets the other kid feel more powerful. It is normal for kids to try to have what's called "social power." When someone is bossy with you or teases you, he or she is trying to have power over you. If you don't stick up for yourself, it gives him or her the power he or she wants. Sticking up for yourself doesn't mean that you have to be aggressive or mean, it just means that you have to talk back to them and show this person that he or she is not making you feel upset (of course, you will be upset and you can tell your friends or family, but not the kid who is teasing you). When you "talk back," you don't want to *ask* this person to stop talking to you like that; rather, you want to *tell* that person that he or she cannot talk to you like that. If the same kid is being rude or hurtful to you, you should role-play with your parent what you can say back.

Finally, kids who are *proactive* and make decisions based on their values (what is important to them) feel better about themselves than kids who are *reactive* and make decisions based on how they feel. For example, if you don't feel like doing homework and decided not to do it, then you are being reactive. But if you don't feel like doing homework, but value going to school the next day prepared, being respectful to your teachers, and being responsible, then you will do your homework. Being proactive makes life a lot cleaner! By facing your fears, you are learning to not be reactive (which leads to avoidance) but to be proactive and let your values guide you!

When facing your fears, it is very important to cheer yourself on and encourage yourself to do the thing you are afraid of. It is very important to know your success as you go along and how you are mastering your worries by facing your fears. Remember that the anxiety tries to get you to doubt yourself (make you feel unsure about yourself), and when you face your fears you are proving it wrong! Tell yourself that you can do it and that you will succeed. Remind yourself that others believe in you—they know that you can do it, too. I *know* that you can do it and I *know* that once you face your fears, you will win the battle against your anxiety!

When facing your fears, try to stay mostly in the order of your ladder. Sometimes you may skip around and this is perfectly fine, as long as you feel ready for it. For example, you may get the chance to do one of your steps, like getting invited to a party (if going to a party is on your ladder), and you might want to take advantage of the chance to do it. Again, this is OK as long as you feel like you are mostly ready to do it. Feeling ready doesn't mean that you will feel no anxiety about doing it; it just means that you are willing to try, and maybe you can picture yourself doing it. Also, most kids find that it gets much easier to face their fears as they go through the steps.

This also is a good time to work on your nervous behaviors that you read about in Chapter 6. Examples of nervous behaviors include asking your mom or dad to tell you a situation will work out alright (called *reassurance-seeking*), clinging, and checking things like if the dog is safe or if the doors are locked. The goal is to get rid of these behaviors. I know it can be very hard to stop doing these behaviors because you are used to doing them, but getting rid of them is part of overcoming your worry and anxiety.

Your mom or dad will help you stop doing the nervous behaviors by reminding you when you are doing them and by not answering questions when you are seeking reassurance from them. They are not doing this to upset you or as a punishment. Your parents' book explains that your mom and dad need to stop telling you that everything will be OK because it makes the anxiety and worry stronger. When your mom or dad tells you that it will be OK (gives you reassurance), it makes you feel better right now, but makes your anxiety and worry worse in the long-term. Instead, your parent will ask you to use your self-talk and relaxation tools to help yourself feel better.

Also, you and your mom or dad may decide to use a calendar to track each day that you don't use your nervous behaviors. For example, at night, Billy would repeatedly ask his mom if he could stay home from school the next day; sometimes she would let him. After coming to therapy, Billy's mom learned that letting him stay home from school was actually making his anxiety worse. His mom then learned to change the way she responded to Billy, and instead she would say to Billy, "You sound nervous about going to school, but you have to go. We cannot allow anxiety to control your life. What can you do to calm down right now?" At first, Billy didn't like this response from his mom, but after a while he got used to it. They used a calendar and every night that Billy didn't ask his mom if he could stay home from school, she would give him a check or a put a sticker on his calendar. He began to see that everything would be fine, even though his mom didn't let him stay home from school. Billy realized that he felt better about himself when he was able to handle his anxiety and worries on his own.

Like Billy, you can get rid of your nervous behaviors and feel better about yourself. Take a minute to think about what nervous behavior you do most often, and tell yourself that you will work on getting rid of it. Getting rid of your nervous behaviors is one of the last parts of overcoming anxiety.

When you take the rest of the steps of your ladder, come up with more replacement thoughts to help you change the way you think about each situation. Try to figure out which thinking mistake you may be making, and then come up with a new, more balanced thought. Remember that you can change the way you think to change the way you feel. The exercise at the end includes a chart that you can use to come up with replacement thoughts for the different steps. Also, don't forget to use the tools in your toolbox; you can look back at the picture of your toolbox in Chapter 6 for a review.

One last note about taking the rest of the steps on your ladder: When kids take a step on their ladder, they don't just do it once and then forget about it. Instead, they continue to do it over and over until it no longer makes them feel anxious or scared. This also is important for you to do. So, once you do something on your ladder, you should continue to do it repeatedly. It soon will become something that you are able and comfortable to do! When you take the rest of the steps on your ladder, you may feel anxious and scared when you do them at first, but I promise that as you continue to practice, it will get easier and easier. Plus, many kids find that they aren't anxious or scared at all when they take one of their steps, and they realize that it was just their anticipatory anxiety talking.

Good luck with taking the rest of your steps!

Chapter 7 EXERCISE

Finish Your Ladder

EXERCISE

Take the next step on your ladder, and then the next step, and so on, until you've taken them all. Remember to go at your own pace, but try to do 1–2 steps each week. If any step feels like it's too much, try breaking it down into smaller steps. Also, you can make additional worry tapes that are specific for certain steps on your ladder.

Don't forget to:

▶ put stickers on your ladder next to the step after you've taken it, and

▶ note what your anxiety level was on the FEAR-mometer.

Change the way you think to change the way you feel! Use steps from your ladder for the chart on the next page (write them under "situation") and write down the automatic thought or worry you have about facing that fear. Then, figure out which thinking error you might have used, and come up with a new, more balanced and accurate thought for your replacement thought. Your parents can help you come up with these new thoughts. When you take each step, try to remind yourself of the replacement thought you came up with for that situation. Good luck!

Situation →	Thoughts →	Thinking Error(s)

Replacement Thoughts:

EXERCISE

Situation →	Thoughts →	Thinking Error(s)

Replacement Thoughts:

Situation →	Thoughts →	Thinking Error(s)

Replacement Thoughts:

EXERCISE

Situation →	Thoughts →	Thinking Error(s)

Replacement Thoughts:

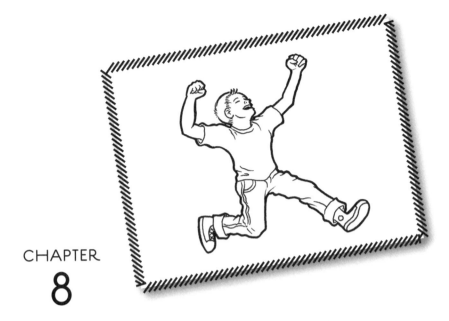

CHAPTER

8

Lessons Learned

Celebrate Yourself

WELCOME to the last chapter of this book! Getting to this chapter is a *great* thing to have done and you deserve a big cheer: "Hurray! Great job! You did it!" You have faced your fears and *won!* In other words: Congratulations!

You deserve a party (and you're going to have one very soon) to celebrate all of your hard work and for trying your very best and overcoming your fears. Now, before you have a celebration with your family, there are two very last things to talk about:

1. What lessons did you learn?
2. How can you handle anxiety and worries if they come up again in the future?

Lessons Learned

So, how did you do it? Let's review what you did to get to the point of facing your fears and overcoming your anxiety.

First, you learned about the three parts of anxiety: body, thoughts, and behavior. After creating your team and team goals and making your ladder, you learned how to work on each of the three parts to overcome your anxiety. To help your body's feelings of anxiety, you learned and practiced:

1. calm breathing,
2. progressive muscle relaxation,
3. relaxing imagery,
4. mindfulness meditation, and
5. yoga.

To help with your anxious thoughts, you learned:

1. how to master your worries (worry tapes, uncertainty training);
2. how to use positive self-talk;
3. about the situation-thought-feeling connection (how you think will affect how you feel, so changing your thoughts can change the way you feel); and
4. about thinking errors and how to change them into healthy replacement thoughts.

Finally, to help with the behaviors part, you learned how to face your fears, one by one, and you did it. You also learned how to get rid of nervous behaviors and worked on those too. Changing the way you think not only changed the way you feel, but it also changed the way you behaved.

By facing your fears, you learned that you can win and overcome your anxiety and take charge of it. Kids who face their fears also often learn that their fears were not as bad as they expected them to be. Once they were in the different situations, they found out it wasn't that bad after all. They learned that they can face their fears.

You also learned that when something difficult or challenging comes your way, you can face it and become stronger as a result. Most kids who face their fears also realize that they feel better about themselves and then their self-esteem improves and becomes stronger. You learned that you can believe in yourself and your abilities to face your fears.

Handling Worry and Anxiety in the Future

Most kids who complete this program and face their fears don't go back to being as anxious and nervous as they were in the beginning. Now that you have read this book and done the exercises, you hopefully are not feeling anxious like you did when you started. But, it is always a good idea to know what to do in case you get a little anxious from time to time, or get really anxious about something different. Well, the best part is: You *know* what to do, because you just did it as you read this book. You can handle any anxiety in the future in the same way that you handled your anxiety during this program. So, even if things come up for you, you can use all of these skills to deal with it and not allow it to become a problem. You are now an expert on how to handle any anxiety in the future.

Let me give you an example: James successfully overcame his fear of snakes by completing this program. More than a year went by without thinking about or worrying about snakes when James went to a birthday party and there was a snake trainer there to put on a show (can you believe it?). Because he had not thought about snakes for so long, when he first saw the huge snake around the neck of the trainer, James suddenly felt a rush of fear. For a moment, he forgot that he was no longer scared of snakes! Then he realized that he knew what to do: He knew that he needed to stay at the party, and actually sat closer to the snake trainer to make it more like he was facing his fears. He also took a few deep breaths and remembered that he could handle this. He reminded himself that he would be OK and that he's done this before so he can do it now. After about 5 minutes, James felt back to normal again. He was calm and felt no fear. James was reminded that whenever he felt anxious, he just needed to use the tools in his toolbox and face his fears.

Like James, you may have some anxiety and worry from time to time. Just do what you have throughout this program, and you'll be fine. Keep this book someplace safe and come back to it whenever you need to. I know that it will all work out for you, and wish you all the best in your future.

Congratulations again and good luck!

Chapter 8 EXERCISE

Celebrate Yourself With a Party and Earn Your Official Certificate of Achievement

EXERCISE

Talk to your parent about the party and who should come to it. Some kids have the party with just their one or two parents, and others invite their siblings, pets, or friends. There is no right or wrong way to do it—the only rule is that you have fun and celebrate all of your hard work and success!

For the Certificate of Achievement, your parent will fill in the information and you can decorate it anyway you like. Have a great party—you deserve it! I am so proud of you!

EXERCISE

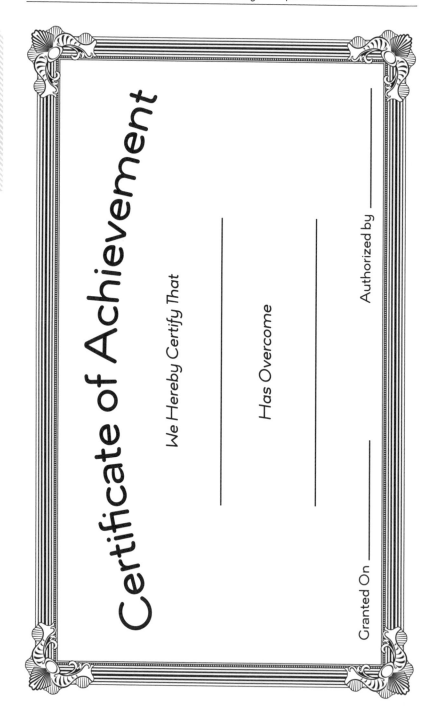

Certificate of Achievement

We Hereby Certify That

_____

Has Overcome

_____

Granted On _____   Authorized by _____

Appendix A
Overview of the Program

This page provides an overview of the program and allows you and your parent to check off when each of the chapters and exercises are completed.

Chapter	Topic	☑ Done
Chapter 1	Anxiety: What It Is and What To Do About It Exercise: Fill in the Bubbles	
Chapter 2	Making Your Team and Team Goals Exercise: Making Your Team and Team Goals	
Chapter 3	Relaxing the Body Exercise: Practice Relaxation	
Chapter 4	Conquer Your Worries Exercise: Self-Talk Note Cards and Worry Tapes	
Chapter 5	Changing Your Thoughts Exercise: Identify and Replace Thinking Errors	
Chapter 6	Changing Your Behaviors: Facing Your Fears Exercise: Facing Your Fears	
Chapter 7	Keep Facing Your Fears and Build Confidence Exercise: Finish Your Ladder	
Chapter 8	Lessons Learned: Celebrate Yourself Exercise: Party and Certificate	

Appendix B

Thinking Errors Quick Reference Page

- *Catastrophizing:* visualizing disaster; thinking that the worst thing is going to happen and feeling like you wouldn't be able to handle it; asking "What if . . ."
- *All-or-Nothing:* thinking in extremes, things are either perfect or a failure; there is no middle ground—it's either one extreme or another; thinking in an inflexible way
- *Filtering:* focusing on the negative parts of a situation while ignoring the positive parts; catching all the bad parts and forgetting about the good parts
- *Magnifying:* making something seem bigger and worse than it really is; turning up the volume on anything bad
- *Shoulds:* rules that you have about how things should be; using the words *should*, *must*, and *ought* to show how things should be
- *Mind Reading:* thinking you know what others are thinking, particularly what they are thinking about you; usually you will think that others are thinking negatively about you
- *Overgeneralization:* taking a single incident and thinking that it will always be this way; something happens once and you think it will always happen this way
- *Personalization:* taking something personally; making it about you when it has nothing to do with you
- *Selective Attention:* paying attention to things that confirm your beliefs about something; ignoring evidence that goes against what you believe about a particular situation
- *Probability Overestimation:* overestimating the likelihood that something bad will happen